Sit, Stay, Grow

How dogs can help you worry less
and walk into a better future

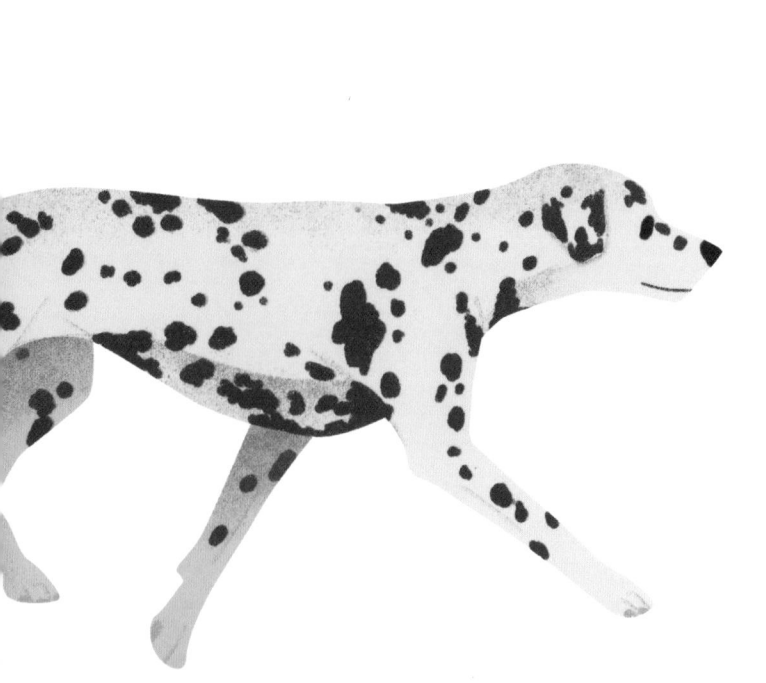

Sit, Stay, Grow

How dogs can help you worry less
and walk into a better future

Angelika von Sanden

Hardie Grant

BOOKS

Contents

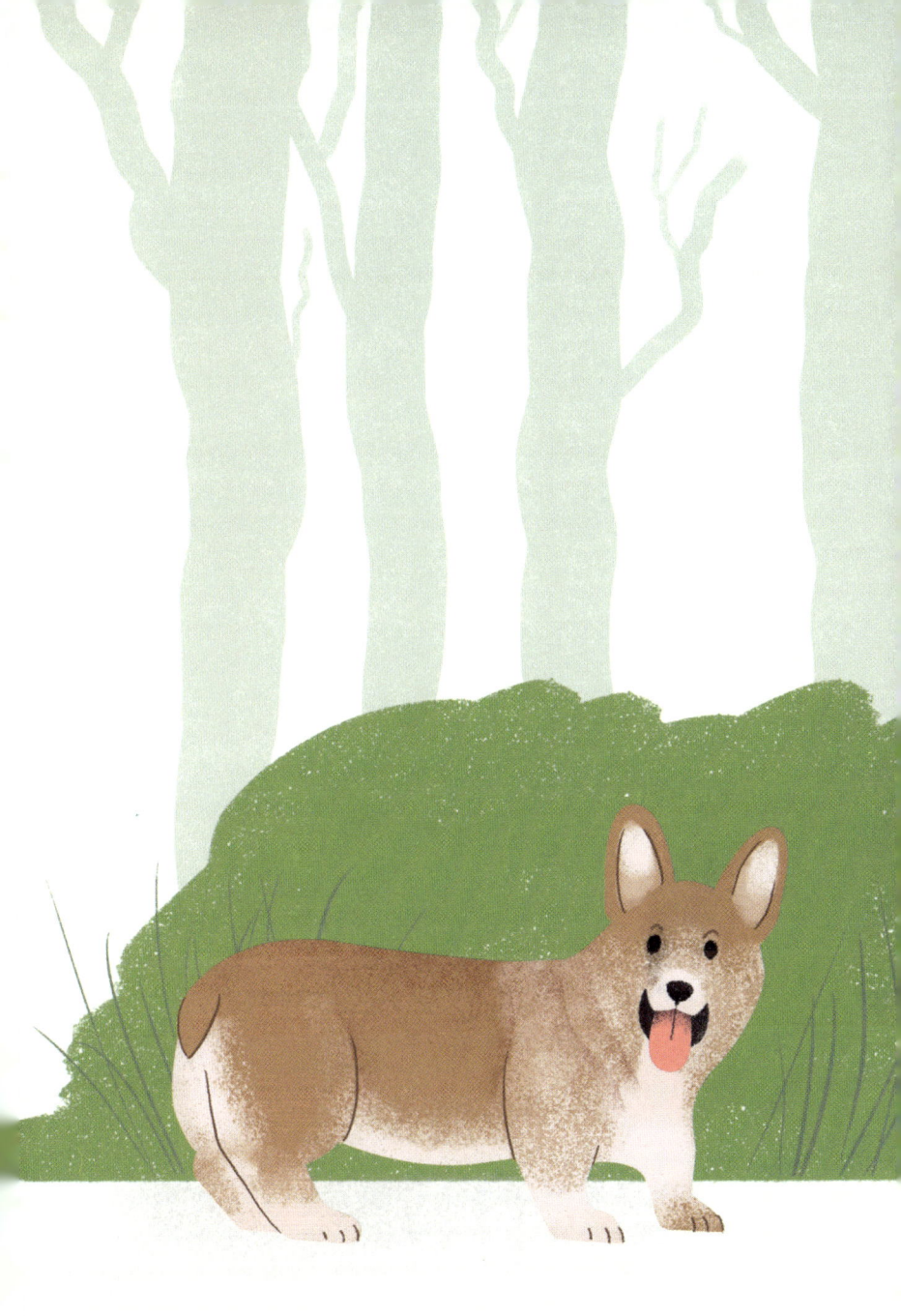

Foreword

I love this book because it's about two of my favourite things; the first being dogs.

Dogs are awesome. I find it mind-blowing that these playful, loyal, loving, trustworthy and truly wonderful companions evolved from ancient wolves. And one of the things this book makes beautifully clear is that there is so much we can learn from them. There's no such thing as a 'dumb dog'. Every canine is a wise and wonderful being, with much to teach us.

Which leads me to my other favourite thing within these pages: Acceptance & Commitment Therapy. Better known by its abbreviation, ACT, this is a scientifically proven approach for transforming your life, through three main methods: developing skills to unhook yourself from

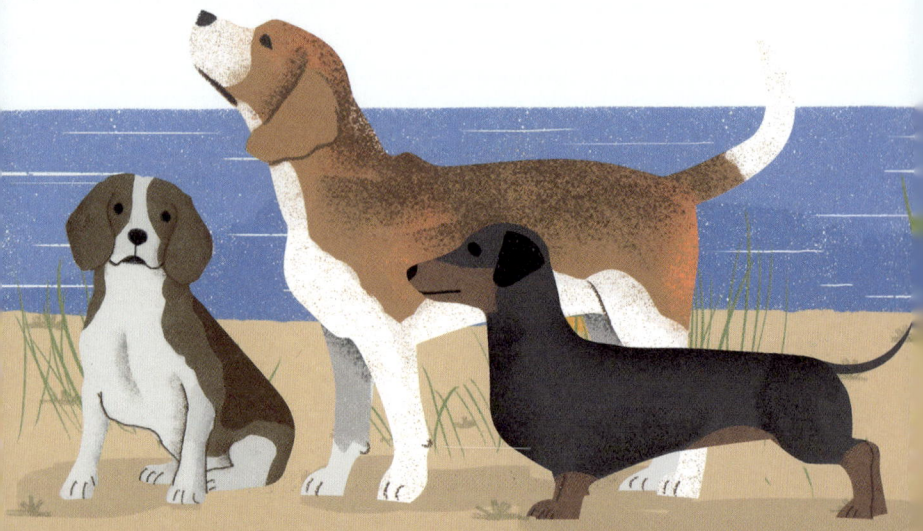

difficult thoughts and feelings; focusing your attention on what matters; and using your core values as a guide for effective life-enhancing action.

Angelika von Sanden has taken the ACT approach and, with a great combination of humour, playfulness and artistry, channelled it into a fun, practical, and easy-to-read book for building a better life. Through the clever use of dogs as role models, she's managed to do this without any of the technical jargon that books on ACT usually include.

Packed full of creative, playful, canine-oriented exercises for developing powerful new psychological skills, this book will help you to handle painful emotions more effectively, unhook from negative thoughts, behave more like the person you want to be, focus on what's important, and engage in what they do.

You're in great hands – enjoy the read!

Russ Harris
Author of *The Happiness Trap* and *ACT Made Simple*

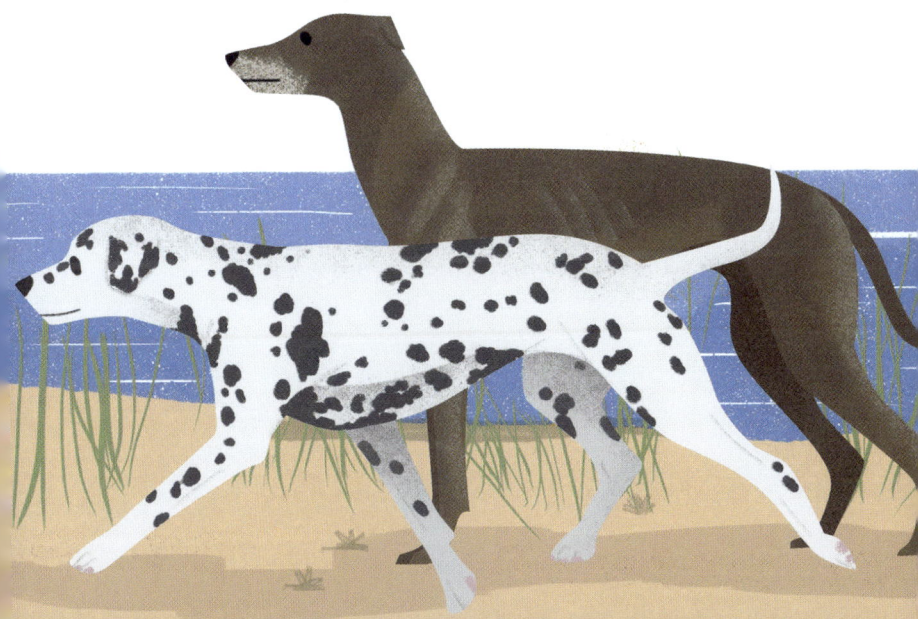

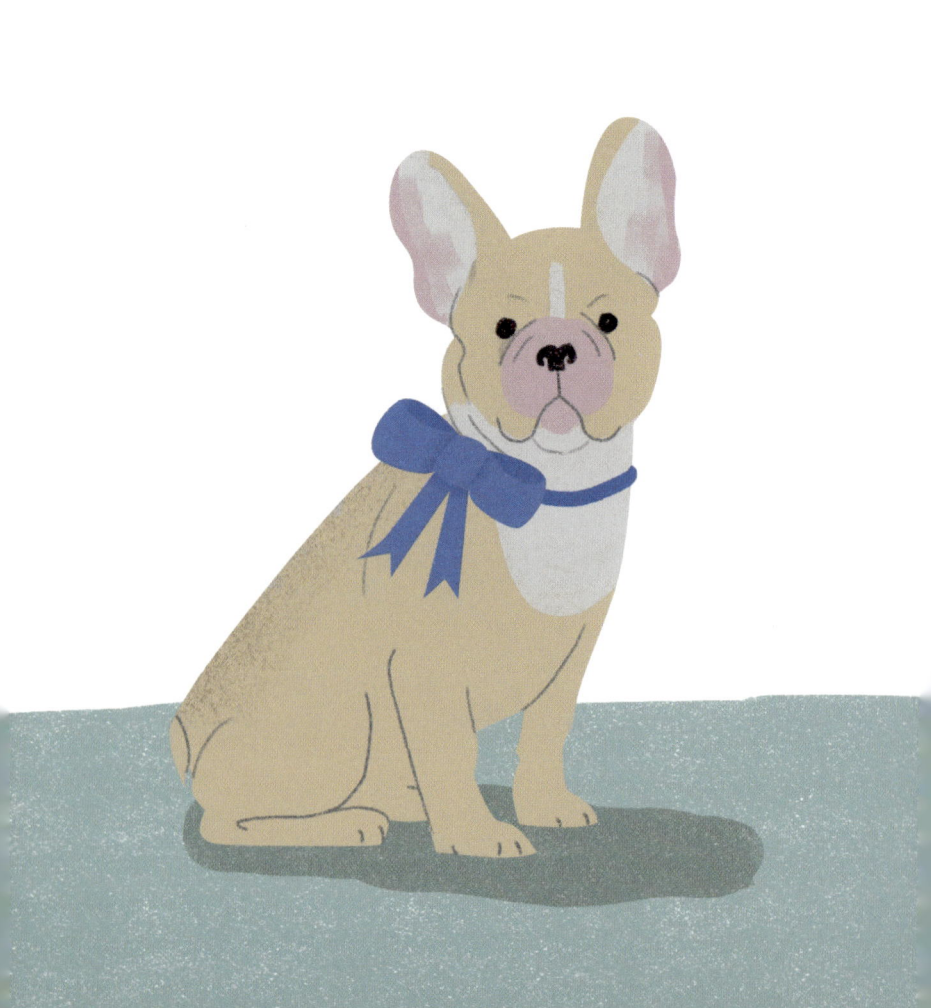

Introduction

The gift which I am sending you is called a dog,
and is, in fact, the most precious
and valuable possession of mankind.

Theodorus Gaza

You know already that dogs are special. Very special indeed! Some describe the furry friend next to their bed as their constant loyal companion or their 'go to' when the world seems unbearable. This book is an attempt to highlight some of their helpful qualities. It will never do the dogs in your life truly justice. They are always so much more …

The first dog I shared my life with was already there, before I was born. The last was called Amigo, the Spanish word for friend. And he truly was one!

Working as a social worker and therapist for decades, I not only heard stories of heartbreaking pain, mind-tumbling anxiety and whole body-paralysing depressive thoughts, but also about the many times dogs were named as the purpose to keep going, the shoulder to cry on and the one steady and non-judgmental being in people's life. The more I listened, the more I understood that animals – often dogs, but also cats, reptiles and once a chicken – are healers, who give unconditional support during hard and lonely times.

Watching dogs during my daily walks, I observe them with their capacity to enjoy life, defend their territory and be fair in their playfulness. I also notice their unique quirks and differences.

Dogs have been around humans for a very long time. They were once a practical addition, helping with hunting, herding and protecting homes. Now, most of them have become companions, friends and fur babies, and an important part of families. In this book, a dog and a person living under the same roof is called a family.

I invite you to take one thought from each of the fourteen chapters in this book with you for a walk and notice what happens when you decide to follow the suggestions. Often, I feel that I am simply putting into words what your dog has already been inviting you to do.

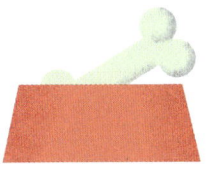

Sometimes I encourage you to go one step further and to do something that might feel uncomfortable, because this may lead you towards a life richer and more meaningful than it feels at the moment.

I've lived and worked in Australia for more than twenty years, but growing up in Germany, I was surrounded by traditional sayings that will stick with me for the rest of my life. As so often happens with sayings, it's impossible to directly translate them into another language, but let me introduce one, which you will come across several times in this book:

'Den inneren Schweinehund überwinden.' An attempt to translate, which does not make sense, would be 'to overcome the inner dog, which looks like a pig'.

What it really means makes much more sense. It is an encouragement to do something that seems hard, knowing that tackling this challenge is about what is truly important to you. It means overcoming the tendency to remain passive and shy away from doing what matters. It matters because it seems uncomfortable or risky. I have no idea where the saying comes from. But I recall many situations where overcoming the inner schweinehund led me to do things that truly mattered, measured by how I would like to be. It led me to walk my dog in pouring rain. Not because I enjoy the rain, but because it mattered to Amigo.

Another example of overcoming my inner schweinehund is right in front of you. Despite so many inner voices telling me that I was unable to write a book, let alone in my second language, I did exactly this. Not because I am convinced that I am good at it, but because it deeply matters to me to share with you what I learned by listening, reflecting and changing myself.

Acceptance and commitment therapy (ACT), the approach I based this book on, invites people to change their way of being. It is not a tactic or a 'how to' with regards to the challenges you encounter; it is an invitation to notice how it feels to be present and choose what matters - to consider yourself and the world around you as part of a larger system. It gives you the motivation and tools to overcome your inner schweinehund and adopt a rich and meaningful life.

Your dog's ancestors didn't need a human companion. They could manage the wild, equipped with their instincts and willingness to survive. But the changed environment means that no dog can live a happy life in a city without a caring human guiding them through the world, which is so different when compared to the experience of the dogs who came long before them.

And just like dogs, your mind needs guidance too! You still have the same instincts, fears and natural tools to survive, but the landscape has changed so much that these are not always helpful in many situations today.

I make no promise of a pain-free or always happy life. For you who loves your dog, you know that on the other side of love there's the fear of loss and pain when the final day comes. I mention this here because honesty is very important to me.

Writing with a knowledge of trauma does not mean that there is nothing in this book that could potentially trigger you. I deliberately avoid all examples describing humans in detail, as humans are the biggest source of trauma. However, if reading or attempting an exercise does trigger you, stop immediately, put both feet firmly on the ground, exhale slowly and inhale in three 'sobs'.

Look at your dog, or a photo of them, and describe what you see. Maybe go for a walk, promising yourself to get back to the book at another time. That you were triggered means that there is something there wanting your attention; a wound waiting to be healed.

Therapy is not the only way forward, but it can be a place to reflect more deeply, be safely supported and to continue to walk in the direction you choose. Trying human therapists until you find one who is most helpful for you is your right. Working with an ACT-trained therapist is one option after or while reading the book. You can also suggest that your therapist works with you and this book. That is your choice. My purpose is to make you aware of your dog's therapeutic skills and how their way of being can support you to be how you want to be in the world.

All dogs' names have been changed to protect their companions' identity. However, Amigo was really named Amigo for a very good reason: he was a loyal friend!

Enjoy the thoughts and take them for many walks. And say 'hi' to your dog from me; I am grateful for what they do for you.

Angelika

This book is not intended to be read in one sitting. I suggest that you read one chapter every few days or a chapter a week, and try to take the same thought for a walk several times. Only then will you notice if the chapter is making a difference or not.

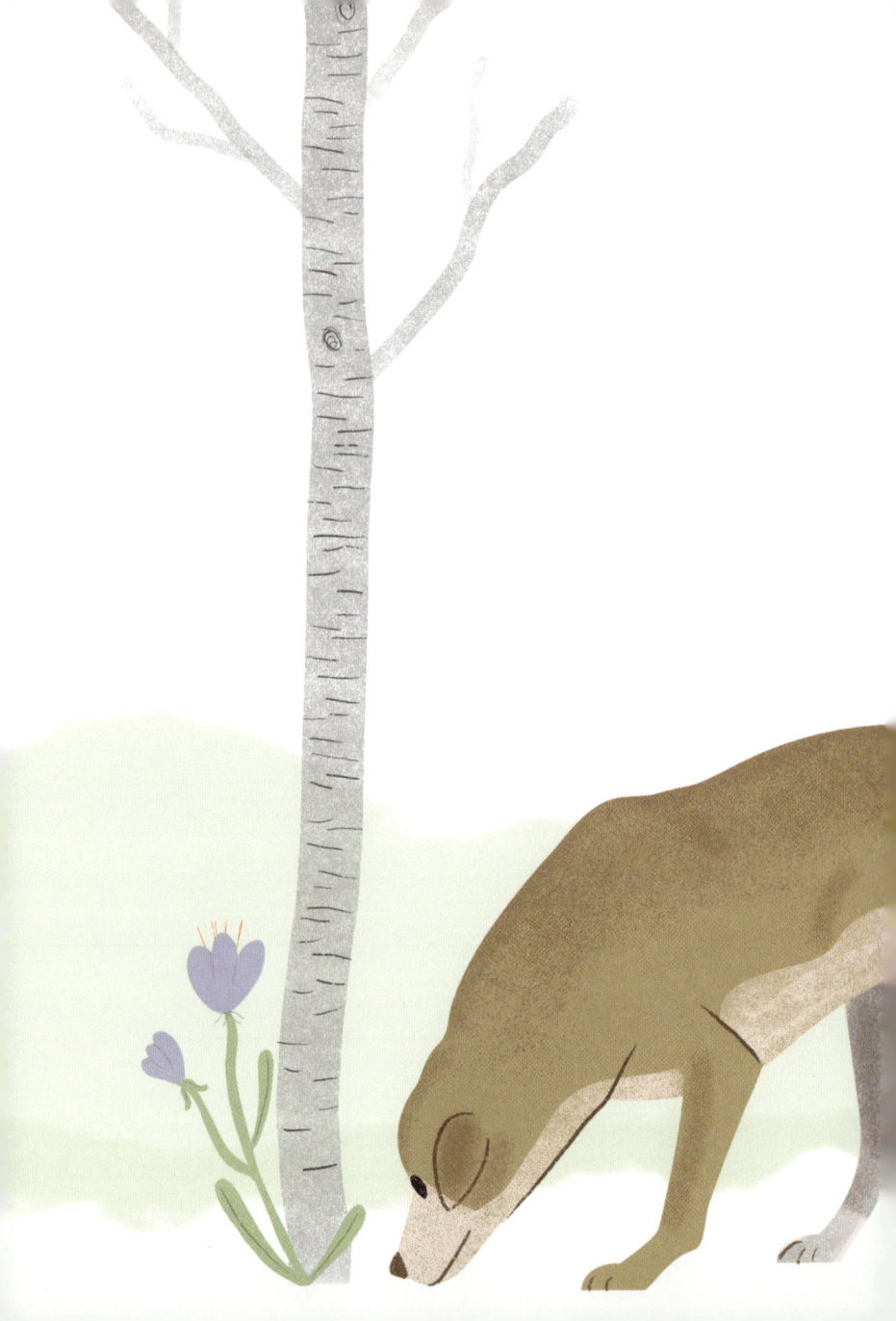

Smell the tree

If you can sit quietly after difficult news;
if in financial downturns you remain perfectly calm;
if you can see your neighbours travel to fantastic places
without a twinge of jealousy …
if you can always find contentment just where you are:
you are probably a dog.

Jack Kornfield

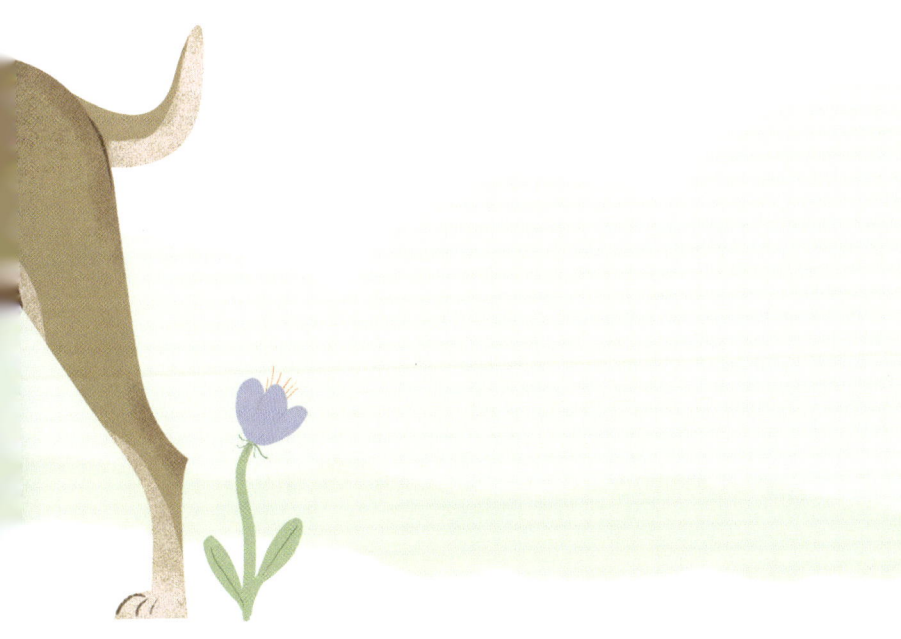

When you start reading this first chapter, your mind might already be thinking about what you should do next or what you should be doing instead of reading a book about dogs and their qualities as a therapist. And maybe your mind already wonders how this could be beneficial. Taking a moment to listen to your thoughts will make you aware that most of them are looking back into the past or trying to predict the future. Your mind might say something like, 'Nothing has worked for me in the past, so I guess nothing will work for me in the future'. But when you observe all there is, you might also notice a thought saying, 'The past cannot predict the future'. If you can, make some room for this thought.

You might be busy with lots of things on your to-do list, and so you hope that this book will not contain another ten exercises you should put time aside for, or another ten things to do with the promise of a happier life.

I have the same hope and wrote this book for people who take their dog for a walk and are willing to take a thought for a walk at the same time.

You will not find any rules in this book or things you 'should' do differently. I do not know how you should best live your life. Whenever I invite you to become aware or give you a choice, I do not do this with the intention of pushing you in the 'right' direction. Shoulds and harsh rules never work in the long run - unless a lot of fear and threats are involved - and have never brought more meaning and happiness to anyone's life. What I would like you to do is notice that with every breath you take, you are also at a point in your life where you have a choice. This awareness is a true alternative to running on autopilot, where things just happen and there's a belief that things are the way they are and nothing will ever be different. I would like to invite you to be aware of options and then choose whatever you would like to choose.

If you make a deliberate choice to stop reading, to eat salad, to stop drinking or to light a cigarette, you can then notice if this is helpful to you or not. If you want a label, this can be called 'acting mindfully'.

But for now, imagine the dog Wincy getting ready for a walk. Wincy knows the time and sits near the front door looking at the leash hanging on the wall and at the door, which will be opened soon. Or so she hopes.

You walk towards the front door, each step followed by Wincy's eyes. There is a hope and an expectation about what might happen next. In this moment, Wincy is an example of mindfulness, being fully present in the here and now.

And as the leash is attached and the front door opens, Wincy strolls out, only a few metres, before stopping and sniffing the tree right opposite the front door. Maybe you have the urge to pull the leash and say, 'Come on Wincy, let's go to the park'.

Today, I would like to invite you to stop with Wincy and look at the tree, as if you have never seen it before. Breathe out and slowly in, and just take a moment. Look at the tree and notice the colour of the bark and the texture. Smell how different it smells outside your house compared to inside. Continue your walk when Wincy tells you to.

Stop a few more times with Wincy on your way to the park and just be in the moment. When your thoughts wander off, be aware that this is what thoughts do. Wincy can teach you lots of things, but you can never be like her. She is a master at being present in the moment. She has reached the highest degree in being. She holds no certificates for having done something amazing or for sitting and passing an exam, yet she knows so much and shares it freely with you – if you are willing to watch and learn.

While it might be a challenge to even stop at one tree and to slow down, it is a great start. Maybe try to do the same at two trees tomorrow and an additional lamp post the day after.

Not all your walks have to be slow, mindful and deliberate. But allowing your mind to settle where you are, and not having to be in the past and the future at the same time, will lower your stress levels and enhance your wellbeing. The benefit is in trying, not in being good at it. Nothing is lost if your mind does what all human minds do: run, walk, jump, or slowly and sneakily hobble away from being present. You win if you commit to try again.

Why is Wincy able to just sniff, while you are thinking about past experiences and things you have to do in the future? Wincy feels safe enough to engage with what is right in front of her nose. People often do not feel safe. So our thoughts go backwards, forwards and often

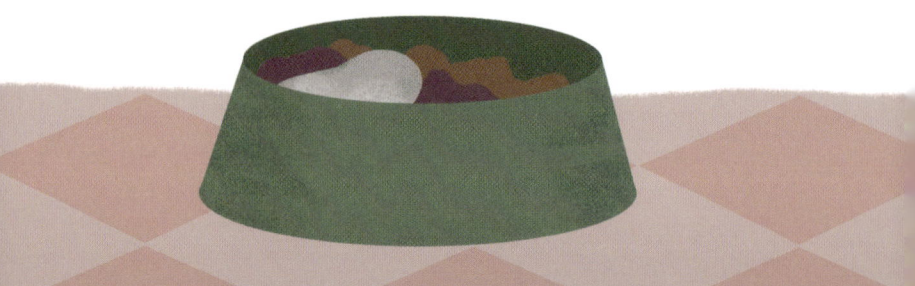

around in circles. Our mind constantly tries to learn from the past and predict the future, hoping to prevent bad things from happening.

These thoughts can become so automatic that you spend time, energy and resources in worrying about things that are clearly outside your control. You might not even notice what is in your control and will consequently 'forget' what you could be doing.

Your worrying mind is an attempt to keep you safe. So, thank your mind for trying to do a good job, while being aware that it has the tendency to go over the top and create a pessimistic outlook on life.

Does Wincy never worry about anything? She does worry!

Coming home from your walk, it is feeding time, and Wincy is still closely enough related to her forefathers, when food was scarce and the one who ate the quickest got most of what was there. Supply could run dry, and hunting was not only a survival skill but one where luck had to be on your side. Wincy's great-great-great-great-grandfathers and grandmothers learned the hard way that eating as quickly as possible was the best decision. So Wincy is still worried that there might not be enough, regardless of how often you tell her or even show her the full cupboard. Words can't land where worry patterns have been formed a long time ago. That's why 'Don't worry, be happy' can only be a song, but not life advice. Watching any dog 'inhaling' food from a bowl shows you what I am talking about.

It did make sense once, but here in your home, with an ongoing food supply, regular feeding times and no other dogs around, it does not make sense at all. Wincy cannot 'just forget' her genetic make-up and force her brain to change to one best adapted to a modern city life, with pet food stores around the corner.

Exactly like it would not work for you if someone told you to 'just worry less' or 'think some positive thoughts'. It does make sense to reflect on the past to learn for the future. It does make sense to try to predict the future. It does make sense to eat quickly and fight for food.

But not always. Not right now, not here, not when you have enough of everything.

Wincy cannot see the bulk dog food package you bought. Wincy needs help to slow down. You can help her and there are ways you can help yourself.

Add some big pebbles to the bowl. Or buy a bowl with some plastic domes. Wincy will have to chase the food with her tongue and will have to slow down. It will be much better for her stomach and much easier to digest food that is chewed and not just swallowed.

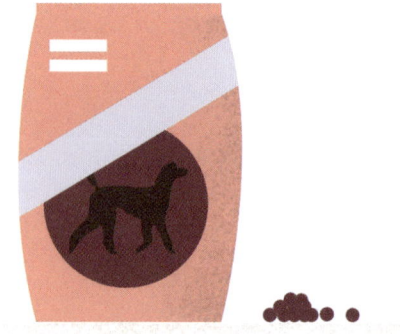

Take a thought for a walk

What could be your pebbles to remind you to slow down? What could help you be in the moment while walking your dog?

Your pebbles could be:
— leave your phone at home
— focus on trees
— notice flowers in gardens
— notice all things red
— watch an ant cross the footpath
— listen to a bird
— watch your dog sniff a lamp post.

 Overcome your inner schweinehund

Overcoming your inner schweinehund is what I call tackling a challenge or jumping over a hurdle. (If this phrase does not make sense, then you have skipped the introduction – many people do, including me. No problem, just go back and read about the German expression and its meaning on page 11.)

You will often find yourself running when you could walk. Thinking many thoughts very quickly when you could be in the moment. You probably often eat fast like Wincy, as if there were wolves about to prey on your food.

There are many reasons why you may do this. Regardless of the reasons, you can challenge yourself to eat more slowly. Smell, lick, taste the food on your fork. Do it again. Or maybe eat a piece of chocolate in front of the TV as slowly as you can. And when it melts on your fingers, lick them as mindfully and joyfully as a piece of good chocolate should be enjoyed.

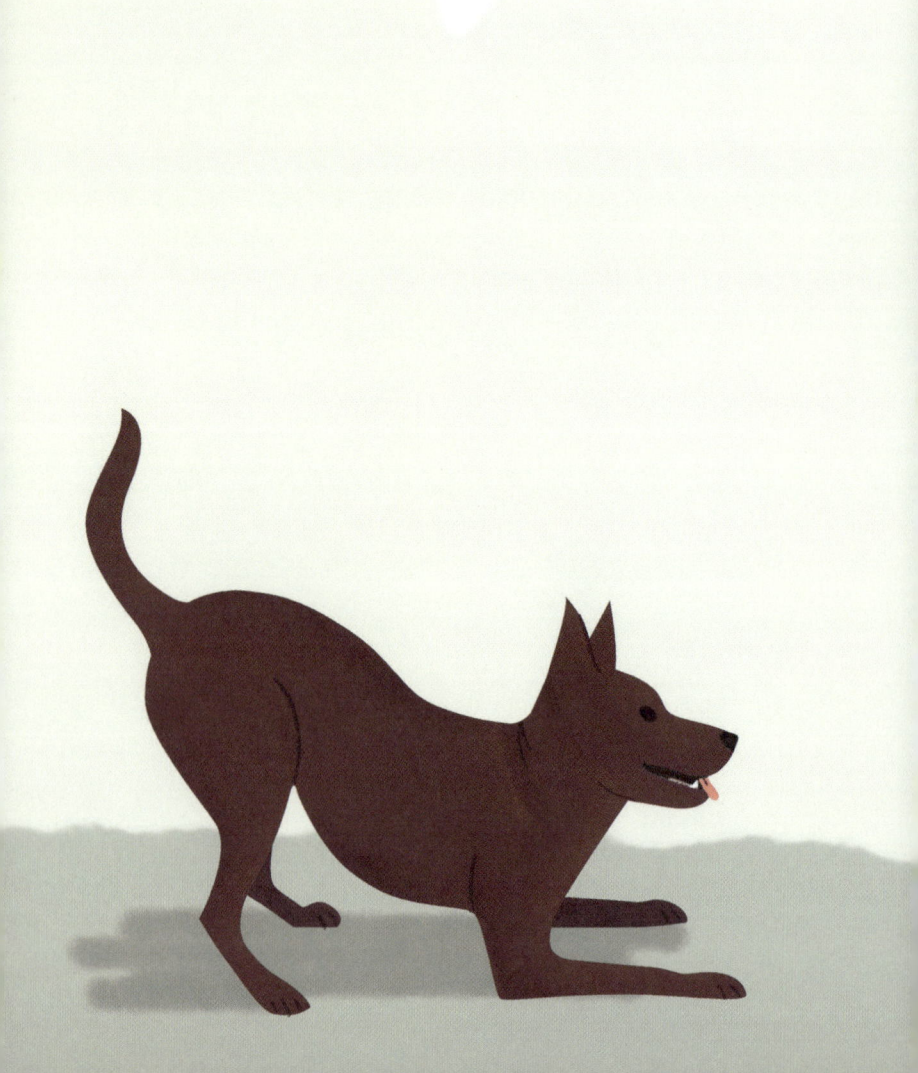

Let's play

I still don't think anything puts me in such
a wonderful mood as playing with Scout.

Haley Young @paws.andreflect

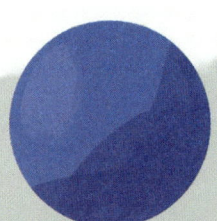

Remember when you played with your dog for the very first time? Take a moment and remember sitting on the floor, holding a toy in front of you and the little fur bundle waddling towards you, wagging her tail and joyfully tugging her teeth into little red Elmo or Rubber Chicken. Since then, you have played with your dog *many* times. Each time she enjoys it as much as the first time. If she doesn't lift her head and follow your hand when you pick up her favourite toy, you would know that something is not right and you might have to see a vet.

On any other day, the moment Amigo entered the off-leash area in our local park, he was eagerly waiting for what would happen next. He had already followed each move I made at home. The moment I picked up the leash, he ran and sat at the front door, and when I opened the cupboard in the hallway, it made him try to look around the corner, without giving up his spot at the front door, to see if I was taking a tennis ball and a thrower with me. If so, his excitement was hard to control! A short stroll to the park, and the moment he was free he would not run off to chase other dogs. He would not go for the person with a pocketful of treats. Sniffing trees seemed totally unimportant compared to looking expectantly at me, hoping that I would throw the ball as far as I could. Chasing the ball and bringing it back was a game he never got tired of. Absorbed in this task, focused on the movement of the ball, trying to predict where the ball would land, and finding and retrieving it was never boring for him. He was only doing one thing at a time. You can observe it with all dogs. They have retained the ability to live in the moment. It might be their secret to contentment and joy.

Amigo, as a kelpie cross, had running, herding and 'working' in his bones and make-up. But he did not need incentives. I never had to ask him to get the ball. It brought him joy – the biggest reward of all!

So much so, that if I did not bring a ball to the off-leash area, he was helping all other dog owners throwing a ball to get it back to them, as quickly as possible. Amigo chased it with amazing speed and before he got old and frail, was only outrun once by another dog, which visibly surprised him. He stopped in his tracks and watched the winner carry the ball back to her owner.

I will admit here that his enthusiasm was not always welcomed by other dog owners, who tried all tricks to encourage their dog to chase the ball too, only to watch them leave it up to Amigo to get it for them. Other dogs engaged in the chase, without any aggression. It was a playful game for the dogs and not about winning.

This is how children engage in play. Before we learned that we should be faster, produce something or be better and try harder, we could all once play like dogs in the park. You were lost in the moment, absorbed by a ball, a little car you pushed from one side to the other, or a crayon leaving colourful marks on a piece of paper. Sound did not have to become tunes, and instruments did not come with music sheets and practice schedules.

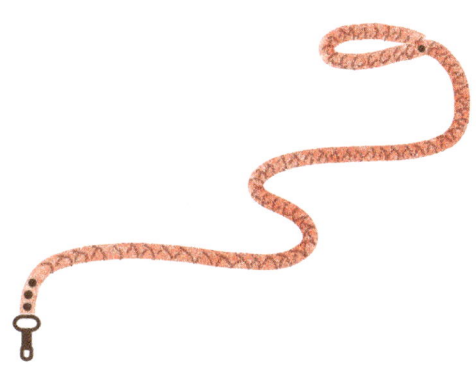

Let's play

While I describe Amigo as the champion in chasing and retrieving balls, he was also a keen swimmer. Easily overtaken by all other keen swimmers, like Alfie the golden retriever and all the muscly staffies at the dog beach, he never gave up and he joyfully jumped in the waves whenever he had a chance.

It is easy for dogs to be playful. They don't have our type of brain, which does what human brains do all the time: judge, compare and having all sorts of thoughts.

Amigo could see that there were dogs swimming more quickly than he was. But this did not make him think, 'I will never be as good as they are, so I may as well give up.' He did not think that because he failed in the dog beach informal swimming competition, he should not even contemplate jumping in the waves again. Of course, this makes it much easier for dogs to experience pure joy.

Humans need to connect to that inner child, to just play.

Adults have lots of thoughts, and we believe, as unhelpful as it can be, that thoughts are the best advisers about what to do or not do. You might not try to play piano because of the thought that you will never be any good at it. And while you might like to try, you might not book the first lesson, because your thought told you that you will suck at it anyway. Most people before you, including me and all who have ever crossed your path, have tried to control their thoughts. Wishing and hoping that without particular thoughts lots of things would be possible. In your mind it might sound like this, 'If only I felt confident, then I would try to …'.

And here's the bad news. You will not be able to get rid of all doubtful thoughts permanently, or indeed any thought at all. You might manage not to have one for a while, by distracting yourself with things like drinking, eating or not eating, watching TV, singing or running a marathon.

My go to is reading. While following a story, I can forget everything else, but the same thoughts will always come back. What if I can never really get rid of these horrible, painful and often nasty thoughts? Does that mean that I can never do or try what I would like to do?

Here is the good news.

Thoughts cannot tell you what to do or who you are. They are random mental events. They just happen. They cannot hold you back, even if it seems like it. You can have a thought, any thought, and you can still do what the thought tells you not to do. Try it out. Notice what kind of thoughts you have and how many of them are coming and going.

Most likely, while reading these last lines, you have not thought about a little white dog. Now think about the cutest little white, fluffy puppy you can imagine. Her eyes are enormous and her tiny pink tongue is licking your hand, greeting you as only a gorgeous creature like this can. And now you might recall a little fur baby bouncing around in the park or a lovely dog belonging to someone you know. But here comes the challenge. Stop thinking about white dogs. Do not think of any dogs at all! Try this for just five minutes – or only three. Do not think about what you were thinking about before!

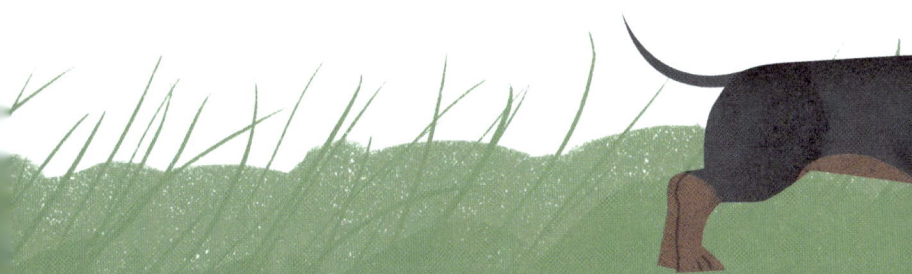

Can you do it? Most people can't. If you succeeded, think about the effort you put in to not think about a dog you saw, a four-legged companion you had or the possible next addition to your family.

Did you have to get up? Walk around? Drink lots of cold water? Switch on the news? Or sing a song? What a huge effort, just to stop you thinking about a random thought I put into your mind.

Think about the effort you make to avoid some thoughts and memories. Not all thoughts are as pleasant as the one I 'planted'. The most dominant memories are the ones that were created with a lot of pain and suffering. They present themselves so vividly that it feels like whatever happened then and there is happening again, here and now.

Regardless of what kind of thoughts your mind comes up with, they cannot tell you what to do. If you just notice them as thoughts or memories, you can have them and start doing what matters. This is maybe a huge and new concept, and it's likely that your mind will immediately come up with a few 'buts'. I don't expect your mind to do anything else. However, you can decide to try it out. And when a thought tells you 'you can't', maybe check if that is true. It might be just a thought holding you back from experiencing pure joy instead of worries.

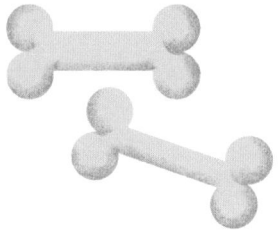

Take a thought for a walk

— When were you last absorbed in doing just one thing,
   without concern for the outcome?
— What else was happening around you?
— What once made you as happy as Amigo chasing a ball
   or swimming in the ocean?
— Do you remember how it felt to be absorbed in the moment,
   so that you stopped comparing your performance with others?
   Many of us have forgotten how that feels.
— What is it you would like to try, regardless of thoughts of 'having
   to get better', 'not being good at it' or 'what a waste of time'?

 ## Overcome your inner schweinehund

Decide to pick one thing you once enjoyed a long time ago, and
do it, regardless of what your mind tells you. The longer ago you
enjoyed it, the bigger the challenge. If your mind goes blank, try
the following activity.

You might think that only children play with sand, leaves and sticks.
Collect some of nature's treasures on your next walk and take them
home to arrange a still life, or just take home one pebble to remind
you of how it feels watching your dog play and be jolly.

One step towards more joy counts much more than a hundred
thoughts of doubts trying to hold you back.

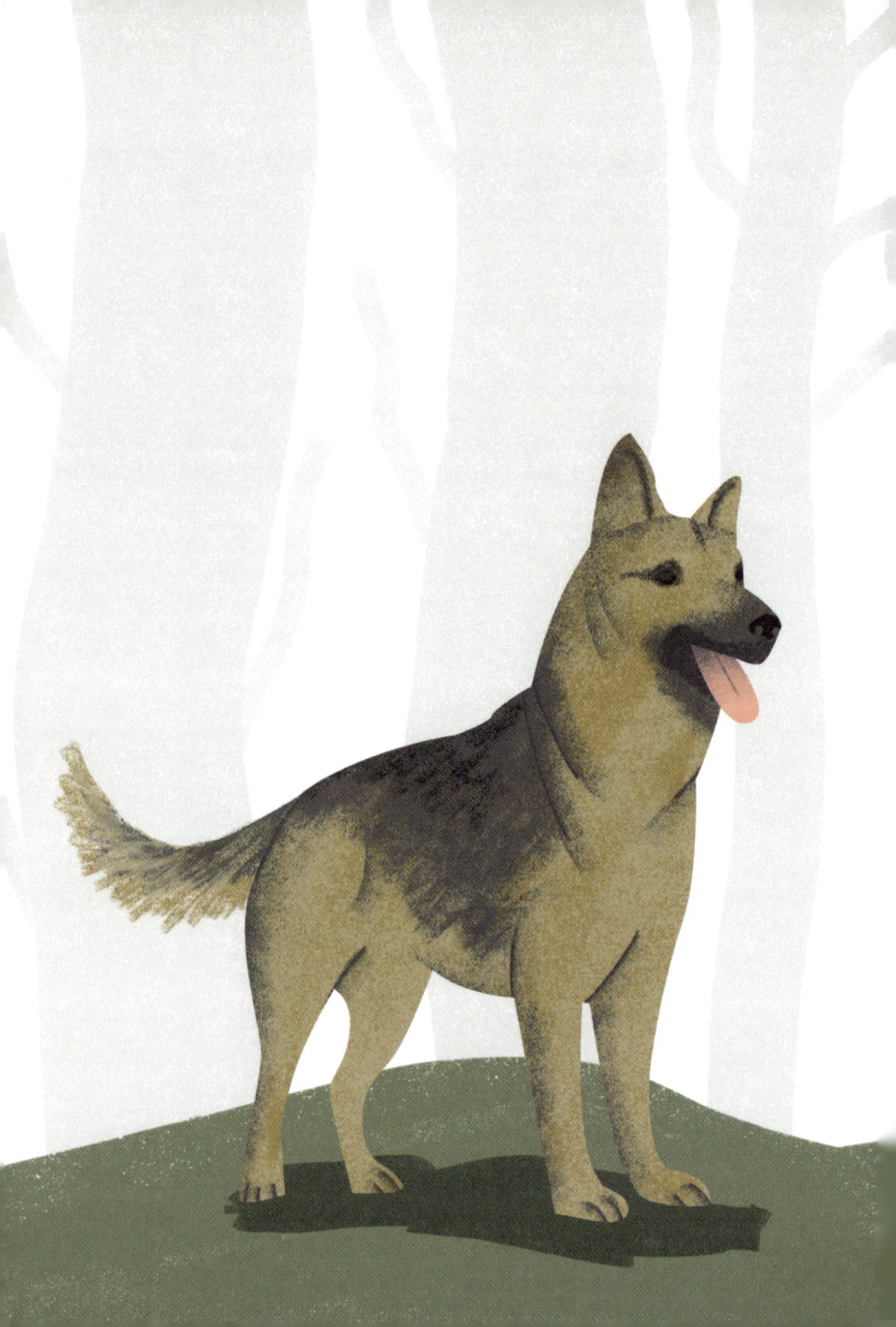

Wild dogs
– wild minds

Even the tiniest poodle or chihuahua
is still a wolf at heart.

Dorothy Hinshaw Patent

When I described Wincy in the first chapter coming home and 'inhaling' her food, I hope that I made it clear that she is not stupid for doing so. It made sense to be quicker than your competitors if you wanted to survive in the wild. The moment Wincy hears the bowl clanging against the kitchen bench, the excitement starts to set in. The tongue comes out and she starts licking, because the saliva is flowing in anticipation of the tasty food her human companion will give her in just a moment. Of course it would be useless to tell her to stop producing saliva.

There has been a long line of ancestors between your fur baby and a wild wolf. Producing saliva before eating helps them to chew and digest. Wincy will drool, even if the food is moist and she could just chew slowly, with no need to get excited beforehand.

What you see are many traits that were once useful in the wild and are still present. You might think that producing saliva might make sense, and sometimes it might, but sometimes not. Either way, Wincy can't stop it from happening.

Here's another example. Amigo was circling on his floor cushion before lying down, although it was equally soft in all its length and breadth. But he was doing what his ancestors did – stepping on the grass to create a cosy place to rest. It is an instinct and it would cost a lot of energy to fight against it, and I guess it would not have made him any happier.

Smurf, a beagle, will sniff for food and more food. Beagles are used at airports to smell out food not allowed to be brought into Australia, and it is a valuable skill and highly regarded. But Smurf also searches for food in bins and is ready to escape and cross busy roads, whenever there is an opportunity, to follow a scent trail. This is unwanted behaviour and can be dangerous, and owners can find themselves giving up on too-eager beagles and, in the best-case scenario, handing them over to border control. It must be a heartbreaking decision and not one I think I could ever make. I would try to put away all food and avoid any places with barbecues, bins and people eating. But I'm not sure this would be achievable or if it would make the beagle's life a happy one.

Smurf's human carer could never imagine giving her away. He has learned to accept that this is what Smurf and most beagles do. He knows that all these traits in dogs, passed on from generation to generation, have a reason for existing and increased their chance of survival.

Some of these instincts can be moderated. Pebbles in a food bowl will slow Wincy down. Training Smurf might lead to some success. However, not all behaviour can be 'untrained', regardless of how skilled the trainer and how clever the dog.

Let me tell you about Inspektor Rex (spelled with a 'k' in the original version). You might already know about him. Inspektor Rex is the main character in an Austrian TV series, later broadcast in many countries, featuring Rex, a German shepherd, as a successful criminal investigator and action hero. When it comes to catching the bad guys – men and women – he's there to help his human partner resolve criminal cases and sometimes survive an ambush. The acting talent of all different canine inspectors during the many years of this series was outstanding. Of course, Rex could follow commands, roll, dig, jump high and wide. He carried lunch to different members of the team and was rewarded with a sandwich himself.

However, when he caught a 'bandit' or attacked the 'thief' in the deepest corner of a rubbish tip, his tail was wagging. Each scene

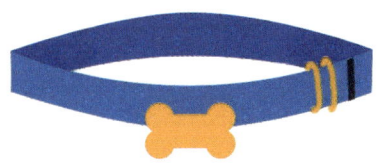

Wild dogs — wild minds

showed either the contradiction of an apparently attacking Rex with a wagging tail, obviously engaging in play fight, or it only showed the front part of Rex, with a growling sound as an add on. Sometimes viewers could see glimpses of the wagging tail and hear the dangerous sounding growling of an aggressive dog.

Nothing can make a dog stop wagging his tail when he feels joy and wants to signal that he is in a good and friendly mood. Even if it does not make sense, according to the film script. Many trainers have tried, as far as I know, but none have succeeded.

There is a piece of wild ancestry in every dog. That's why I chose the quote at the beginning of this chapter. And not only in dogs; we carry our genetic make-up from generation to generation too – habits, traits, thoughts, vigilance and physical responses – even if they do not all make sense in the world we currently live in.

All human beings have experienced anxiety or fear when it wasn't helpful to feel that way, and when it was not justified by what was actually happening. There is a children's book in Germany called *There is a crocodile under my bed*. For the child about to go to bed the fear is real, and the verbal reassurance that it's not true can only give short relief, or none at all.

We all have our crocodiles under our beds. Anxiety is a highly unsettling emotion: a bundle of terrifying thoughts, a raised heartbeat and, at times, a shortness of breath. How on earth has this uncomfortable, or even painful feeling you might experience in the middle of the night ever been helpful?

Let's consider for a moment what your life would look like without anxious thoughts. You would enjoy just being. Sleeping at night, loving deeply, caring without expecting anything in return, breathing in and out while whistling a tune or singing your favourite song (without a thought about your inability to sing). Wouldn't this be wonderful? Absolutely and without a doubt. But only for a short while, and then the blissful moment may turn into bad news.

Because there could be a crocodile under your bed, or a tree falling on your head, or a tiger could have a dinner in your little campsite. Without doubts and fears and a whole bunch of 'What if…?' questions, you and I would not exist. Because your forefathers and foremothers would have joyfully eaten all the fruit they could find, including the poisonous deadly nightshade without caution. Campsites would have been built in crocodile-invested wetlands.

Maybe some would have lived in areas without crocodiles and where all the fruits and vegetables were nutritious and led to even better health. But without looking, checking, warning others and their children, they would have taken a bite from a sweet apple without considering that swallowing a wasp can end in death. So regardless of what kind of idyllic scenario you imagine, in real life there are dangers you need to be aware of. We go further, and tend to try to predict the unpredictable.

Just as Inspektor Rex cannot stop wagging his tail, you are equally unable to stop the anxious and worrying thoughts that are preparing you for action. This certainly makes sense when you encounter dangerous wildlife. Unfortunately, in the middle of the night in your suburban bedroom there is no action to take to make your world a safer place.

Anxiety is a combination of worrying thoughts and physical symptoms. It can start in the mind, with a scary thought, an elaborate horror story or a few thoughts on constant repeat. It can feel like you have an inability to 'just stop' or control what is happening inside your body and mind. Both are so closely connected that it is often near impossible to be aware of them separately.

After the thoughts begin, nearly immediately, physical symptoms follow. These can be a raised heartbeat, shallow breathing, an increase of stress hormones, a clenched jaw, hunched shoulders or shortness of breath, which increases the heart rate and signals to the brain that something might be wrong. If the brain can respond with, 'No problem, I know why this is happening. You had three cups of coffee and you are chasing little Goofy across the beach', then you can think in response, 'Ah, that's it! Thank you, brain - that makes sense.'

But what if you can't explain it? Then the thoughts and physical symptoms can feel dangerous and you might try to think your way out of it or you might try to do whatever it takes to feel differently.

I do not give examples here, as I know examples can trigger what I am talking about. But if you take a moment, you will remember a night or a situation when your thoughts circled around in your head and could not find an exit, repeating again and again the same thing, while your body responded with panic.

You might have tried to command your brain to relax or to divert attention to something else, such as watching TV, listening to music, eating something delicious, taking medication or just ignoring the carousel in your mind. All of this might be good advice and work for a while. That is, until the thoughts come back and you are on the carousel again, without the ability to jump off or stop it.

You might have put even more effort into trying to get rid of those painful thoughts by calling them stupid, and by reading books promising that you can change your thinking. Or you might have tried to become an expert in meditation. And these strategies could have worked sometimes, but the thoughts came back.

If your life's circumstances have changed maybe it's a different story, but it will still have the same intensity, with your mind asking 'What if …?' and not providing any calming answers.

Now consider a new 'What if?'. What if you could learn to live with your wild mind as it is, like Wincy's and Smurf's human guardians do with the 'wild part' in their beloved pups?

Smurf's owner has tried to change what can be changed. He walks him away from public barbecues and does not start a conversation with a person eating a sausage roll. He tells Smurf there will be enough food at home and that there is no reason to dive into bins. Yet in an unsupervised moment, Smurf will do what your mind does in the middle of the night. She will dive into the bin, just like your mind dives into the rip of thoughts that stop you swimming to shore.

The advantage you have, compared to Wincy, Inspektor Rex, Smurf and Amigo, is that you are able to take a two-legged perspective. You can notice what is happening, name it, observe your mind and your body, and help both.

Being caught in anxiety has a lot of similarities to being caught in a rip. Growing up in the south of Germany, I didn't have the chance to witness the enormity and power of an ocean before moving to Australia.

Amigo was still a young dog and not fully trained (was he ever?) when I went with him on a holiday to a beach not far from Melbourne. Ninety Mile Beach is, as the name suggests, a seemingly endless stretch of sand with powerful waves and often strong winds. Amigo was clearly enjoying himself, running, digging and jumping in and out of the shallow water, as waves rolled in over the sand. There were no other people in sight and no designated swimming areas with lifesavers on duty.

Amigo chased seagulls that flew up for a few metres, shrieking, before settling on the sand again. But one of them landed on a wave close to the beach. The next thing I saw, and what still makes my heart stop for a beat, was Amigo running towards the floating seagull and being carried away from the shore towards the open sea. I screamed from the top of my lungs while waving frantically. I could not make out if he was paddling away from me or if a rip was taking him out.

There was nothing I could do but helplessly watch how the distance between us grew while he bobbed up and down, in sight for a moment and then gone again. It seemed like time stood still and minutes stretched to eternity, as Amigo was floating, paddling, fighting against and then carried with the waves, by now parallel to the beach.

These challenging minutes of my life ended when he miraculously reached safe ground again, about 200 metres away from where he went

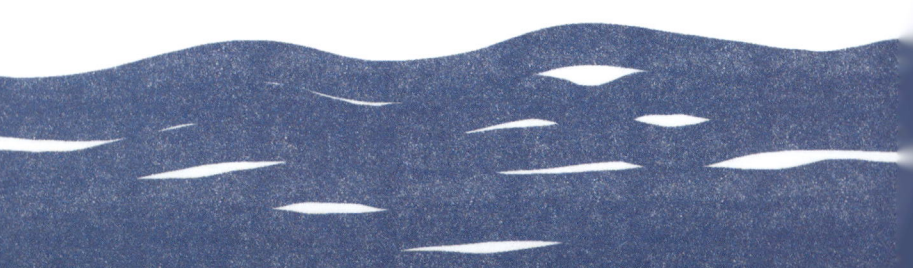

in. Exhausted, but otherwise fine, he shook his little body, not only
to dry more quickly but most certainly to shake off the stress he had
just experienced.

This memory is ingrained in my brain. When I think about it now, it feels
like a watered-down version of how it felt on the day. I still get the sense
of the helplessness I felt then and there.

Experiencing anxiety or panic feels like being caught in a rip. Regardless
of the effort and attempts to swim ashore, you fail and fail again.
Swimming lessons, books about swimming techniques or strength
training do not make you able to swim against a strong rip. It quickly
becomes exhausting and soon dangerous.

Anxiety and panic is the rip you find yourself in, sometimes in the
middle of the night without any apparent reason. Sometimes it happens
during the day in situations you dislike and fear, and would rather avoid.

With the advantage of your two-legged perspective, you might have
learned something I first heard of in Peru, forgot a short time later,
and now living near the ocean get reminded of on a regular basis.

— Do not try to out-swim a rip
— Do not focus on the shortest distance to the shore, attempting
   to swim against a rip
— Do stay afloat and breathe.

What is helpful in a rip is also helpful while in the grip of anxiety
or panic.

D.O.G. RELAX

To guide you through this exercise, I will think about Amigo, my companion for many years. Fill in the name of your four-legged therapist.

You will think of ...

Even better, sit next to ... on the floor, feel how the floor supports you and put your hand on the dog.

or

Sit on the couch, feel your feet touching the floor while your hand rests on your dog next to you.

DESCRIBE

Describe your thoughts to your four-legged therapist. Let them hear all about your many worries. Notice the huge number of thoughts filling your mind. Complete one or more of the following examples:

— I am having the thought that ...
— My mind is saying to me ...
— My mind is calling me ...
— The pain is in my ... and it feels like ...

OBSERVE

Often you have the same few thoughts in slightly different variations. When I notice that, I know that I am caught in a rip. I will name the main thought, like the headline of a story, or I will label it with a self-adhesive sticker saying, 'Here is the old story of ... again'. If it is difficult for you to come up with an example of an old story, ask yourself:

— How often have I described myself as ...?
— How often have I had the thought that I should have
   or could have ...?
— How often have I wondered, 'What if ...'?
— How often have I thought, 'If only ...'?

All these thoughts have become stories your mind repeats. It is highly unlikely that it is your first time in a rip of thoughts and emotions.

Observe your thoughts, stories, physical sensations and emotions moving alongside each other.

GO WITH IT

Go with it and let it be. While sitting on the floor or the couch, feet on the ground, hand on ...'s side, allow the thoughts and feelings to be there. Just as your dog is there next to you. Be where you are, be with what is.

Your heart might beat faster and you might feel scared. It does not make a difference to your thoughts. If you wish them to be different, it just makes you feel worse.

Allowing thoughts to be there, making room for the rip to roll, does not mean liking it or not being afraid. The pain is real and so is the fear. Yet the fight against the rip will not lead to changing its strength. Even if you swim with all your might against it, the rip will still carry you in its direction. Going with it is coming to terms with the rip being stronger than you.

There is only one choice you have in that moment of panic and despair. It is to choose how to be with what you cannot change. So you could say, 'And here I am caught in the rip of my thoughts that are throwing me around. I have lost distance between me and my thoughts. Nothing has worked so far to keep me permanently out of these rips, so I will be with it, floating, knowing that each wave will eventually hit the shore'.

When you are in pain, your dog does notice. Often she will come closer and keep still.

... is just there. And that is a lot. Notice ... next to you.

While allowing all there is to be, your hand rests on her side. You can softly say, 'You are here with me and I am here with you. Right now, we float in a rip but we are still alive'.

RELAX

With your hand still on her, listen and feel her breath going in and out.

Now deliberately breathe out, letting all the used air out of your lungs.

Sigh, like many dogs do before collapsing on their mat for another nap.

Slowly and with 'effortless effort' let the fresh air flow into your lungs.

...'s breathing rhythm is too fast for you, but it is a steady rhythm of in and out and you can find your own. While continuing to breathe slowly and with intention, let your attention wander to your hand on ...'s side. Feel the soft fur where the back meets the belly. Talk to yourself the way you would talk to her when she is afraid of a thunderstorm.

Use the same kind of words and tone you would use for her going through a painful procedure at the vet.

Notice her hair has many different colours or play with the curly locks or the hair around the paws.

... is relaxed beside you.

You can then start to check how relaxed you are:

Smooth out your forehead, unclench your jaw, roll back your shoulders, relax your arm and hand, and now your other arm and other hand.

Softly touching ...'s side, feel your legs, release your calf muscles, notice your feet touching the floor and wiggle your toes.

Start from head to toes again. Repeat as often as you want to, until you feel a sense of calm. Don't let your restless puppy-like mind distract you. Just gently call it back to the task.

You have just discovered a way of floating in a rip with a tool that will always be with you, your breath. You have experienced that no feeling is bigger than you are.

When you are calm, now or on another day, you can try to figure out what your 'natural' response is when you are caught in a rip.

— Are you determined to swim against the rip with all your muscles and willpower? Are you angrily making others responsible for your situation?

If yes, then your response is 'fight'. Often, but not always, this energy can help you to change things you can change, but this response is unhelpful when you are trying to change what cannot be changed.

— Are you investing all your resources in finding ways out? Running away and ending the situation you are in, regardless of the price you pay?

If yes, then 'flight' is your preferred response. While running away can be lifesaving in some circumstances, you will not be able to outrun your thoughts and memories. Of course you can use this strategy when it really is helpful.

If you feel you have no energy left, do not give up. To collapse or flop is a way your nervous system responds when it is overwhelmed with what is happening in your mind and body. It feels intensely helpless but you can help yourself by going through the D.O.G. Relax exercise.

Remember how you taught your newest family member to come back to you? You might have asked an experienced dog trainer for tips, but it was up to you to practise with your dog. Equally it can be beneficial for you to connect with a mentor, coach or therapist, or to call a helpline, while being aware that it is still you who needs to practise to see change.

— Do you hope to be rescued by someone stronger? Would you do anything for the promise that someone can take the thoughts away or change them?

Your 'cry for help' expresses how lonely you feel in that moment. Yet if a magician could come and do all you hope for, it would not make you stronger, more independent and a person your dog feels safe with.

There is nothing wrong with wishing things to be different, with trying to avoid what is painful and moving away from what does not feel good. However, all of this is not possible when caught in a rip, and it is not helpful to spend time and waste energy wishing.

Helpful is to describe and observe. Helpful is to go with it and to relax.

Helpful is to use your breath, to notice … next to you and to name three things you can see. What can you hear? And what else? Listen to the sounds around you or listen to the silence. Is there anything you can smell? Is there a smell you like or one that you dislike? (Oh, those dogs don't have any shame when it comes to farts.)

And unless you have to jump up and open a window, take another few seconds to just be and breathe.

Make this exercise your own. Change the wording if you like and practise in calm waters. Lifesavers at the beach are not trained for emergencies by quickly reading a protocol about what to do in a rip when someone needs to be rescued.

Practise - not reading about it - leads to a deeper learning and the higher likelihood that it stays with you and can be recalled when needed. You cannot learn when stressed, so picking up this book and quickly going through these pages when the waves are high will most likely not work. Preparing now for when things get tough makes much more sense.

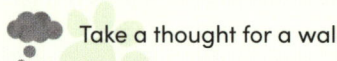

Take a thought for a walk

Notice a slightly unpleasant thought you have often. Not one that is too triggering.

Say to yourself, 'Here is that thought again'. Notice the emotion going with that thought. Don't debate if that thought is right or wrong, or how much you dislike the emotion. Just notice and see the thought for what it is; an attempt by your brain to warn you and help you to stay safe. Silently say to your brain, 'I get it. You just do what you were created to do, trying to keep me safe'. Just like Wincy's brain is telling her to eat as fast as she can. Even if that is not the most helpful advice now. This is what brains do.'

When you have a moment go back to your D.O.G. Relax exercise on page 40. The more often you practise the steps, the more prepared you will be to float and let the rip take its course.

Overcome your inner schweinehund

It is a very strong inner schweinehund that constantly repeats, 'If you would only then you would think and feel differently'.

Overcoming this inner schweinehund will be a lifelong task. Just like taking showers to stay clean.

Or to use another metaphor, the thoughts are there, like a background radio program in some supermarkets, interrupting the music to advertise the latest specials. You get to choose if you stop to listen with all your attention or if you decide to continue with your shopping, not forgetting your puppy's favourite treat.

Overcoming this inner schweinehund means making deliberate choices about what to do – regardless of what music, thoughts or feelings are 'playing' in the background.

It can, for example, mean to take Bodhi for a long walk along the river, while thinking that you would rather like to spend the afternoon on the couch, watching another movie. It is not easy and often uncomfortable.

The next chapter is about how to practise walking towards achieving your goals. What you embrace in puppy training can be helpful for you and improve your life too.

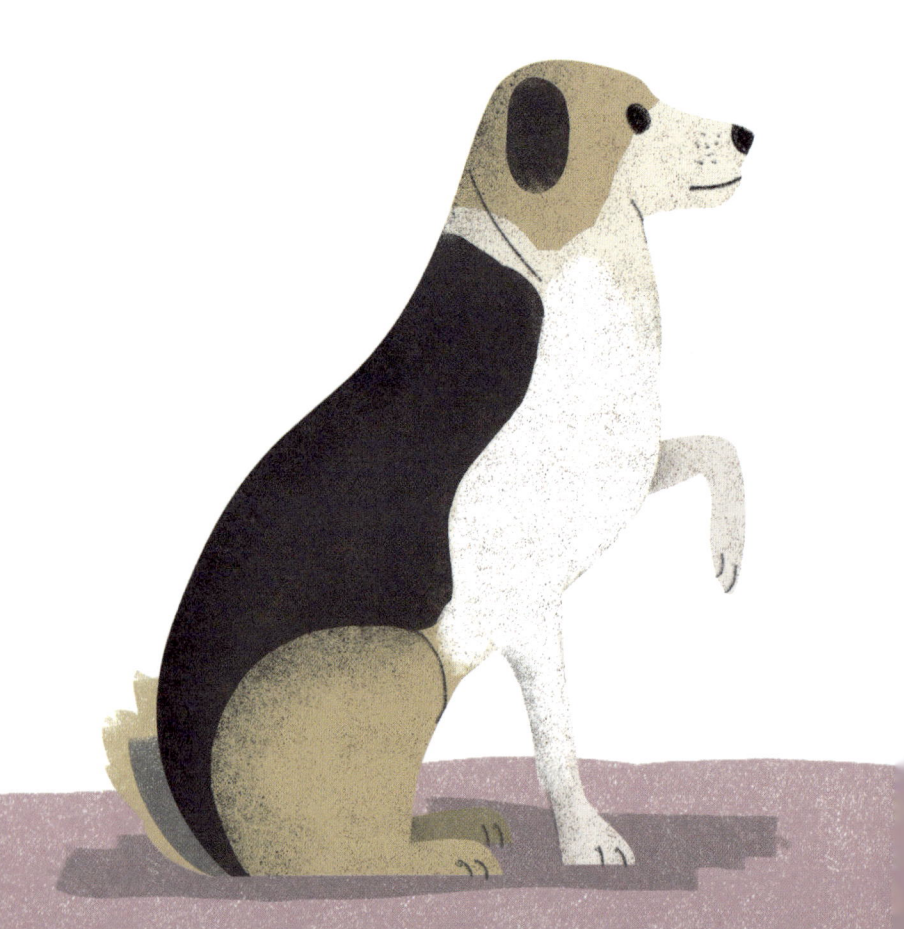

Puppy training

Aligning with our values includes not only
what we do and why we do it
but how we do it.

Joan Halifax

When you held your puppy for the first time, when you saw her running towards you, wagging her little tail, you most likely felt a sense of joy and a warm feeling that you don't experience every day. That's why it would be great to celebrate the moment your puppy entered your life more than once a year. What if you take a few minutes now to feel how you felt then? It can be like going on a short retreat or entering an oasis in the desert - a moment of joyful being.

When you arrived at home on that special day, it was difficult to take your eyes off this little ball of energy. Watching her collapse and sleep, seemingly with the sweetest dreams, was a source of pleasure.

As soon as you could, you took her on her first walk on a leash. Chances are that she did not like it. It did not make sense to her to be harnessed and not able to run free. She wanted to greet everyone on the footpath, and smell and lick each dog. But it made sense to you to keep her on the leash, knowing that she would not be safe if you let her run wherever her little legs took her. You knew you could not give in and let her off the leash.

The first words Amigo heard and soon understood were 'wait' and 'not now'. His energy seemed endless and so he pulled on the leash, wanting to run free and enjoy his ball game. It would have been easier to give in, but of course it meant that he could have been hit by a car while crossing the road to the park. It did not even cross my mind to give in when the risk of harm was so obvious.

It doesn't matter if you choose to join puppy training classes or train your dog alone, patience will still be a main requirement. To me, successful dog training is when the dog follows commands, not out of fear, but out of loyalty and playfulness, and with a desire to achieve something because it feels good. Vision Australia once had an open day, and a dog trainer with a group of kelpies presented his crew. Kelpies are highly energetic dogs, searching for jobs wherever they go. I went to his presentation hoping to pick up some ideas for

Amigo, a kelpie cross, as he seemed unable to do what other dogs did easily during puppy training. I was frustrated to see how Missy the labrador followed her owner, being rewarded with a piece of chicken liver. Prince, a toy poodle, walked perfectly on a loosely hanging leash because, again, chicken liver was waiting as a reward.

I went to puppy training with a pocket full of chicken liver and was loved, sniffed out and followed by a few dogs off leash. Amigo, off leash, had other interests; he started to herd smaller dogs who tempted to stray too far. He was on the lookout for anyone with a ball, scanning for ball throwers or balls hidden in hands or pockets. Chicken liver was not an incentive for him.

At the open day, the trainer's patience with the dogs was what stood out for me. It was not a perfectly polished performance but a demonstration, showing how he worked with dogs at different levels of training. There were the older ones, perfect at climbing, jumping and running through an obstacle course. Then there were some 'teenagers', who followed some commands and then found other things more interesting. Only one was a 'beginner', entertaining the audience with cuteness and not much sense about what was expected of him.

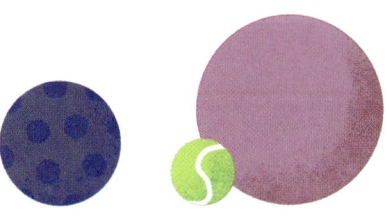

Puppy training

Three things stayed with me: patience, persistence and setting realistic goals. Regardless of what his dogs did or did not do, the trainer stayed patient, repeating commands in a calm voice and directing them towards the next step. While most will agree that this is the best approach to puppy training, I thought about his potential fear that things might get out of hand during his presentation, and his potential frustration if the leading dogs 'stuffed up'. I imagined his struggle with his own expectations about how things should go on the day.

Being patient is not easy.

It means that he lived what he was trying to teach the dogs, and he could not just pretend. As all dog lovers know, dogs pick up on moods and impatience cannot be hidden from a sensitive dog.

My patience and perseverance taught Amigo some patience on the way to the park. The calm repetition of 'wait' and 'not now' helped him to slow down, knowing that the park was not far. It is often said that dogs choose us, based on who we are and what we like and what we need to learn. Amigo was a perfect example. Highly energetic and up for walks, just as I like it. However, he was also a mirror image of

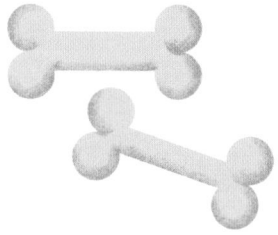

me in his struggle with patience. So what stayed with me from that day was that we cannot expect patience from our dogs if we are not demonstrating patience with them. Sounds simple and it is simple, but not easy! Especially for a fur mum like me – patience and slowing down is not part of my natural make-up.

Persistence means that you continue with a course of action, despite difficulties or opposition. Persistence means that you will change your strategy if it turns out that it is the wrong one. One of the training elements in puppy school was to teach the dog to sit. All the other dogs – and none of the kelpies – did so, getting rewarded with favourite treats. As they sat more often, more quickly and on command, they were rewarded with chicken liver. Not so Amigo. Feeling like a puppy training class failure, I asked the kelpie trainer if there was any other trick he used, rather than tasty rewards. To my surprise, he told me that food was generally not a reward he used with his crew. He taught me that if I looked at Amigo, told him to sit down and kept eye contact, he would follow the command and wait for the next command to come. And it worked! After a few attempts, I carried home the invisible trophy of 'best-sitting dog' after the next training session. Looking at Amigo while he sat down had a calming effect, but only if I focused on him and he on me. He could soon also stay on the spot and let me move away, waiting patiently until I released him and allowed him to run towards me. And if this sounds a bit like bragging – yes, it is. I thought I needed to tell you all this first, before I let you know his limitations. He was the best dog and he had some quirks, like we all do.

Setting realistic goals means that you do not expect Prince, the toy poodle, to jump over a two-metre fence. It also means that you do not expect Bailey, a rescue greyhound trained to chase fluffy fur balls, to get along with a neighbour's cat peeking over the fence. It is more difficult to define realistic goals when dogs 'should' reach certain standards and struggle to do so.

Prince is off the hook in this regard. Nobody will expect him to climb fences. Bailey, however, might be eyed with more scepticism in the dog park. People might wonder why he could not be properly trained so that he could be off leash, without potentially chasing small fluffy dogs.

Amigo, or rather I, feared being judged, as some might assume that a well-trained dog would not chase other people's balls. Once someone even said to their dog, 'We don't play with this kind of dog, do we?'. I still believe that the dogs were fine. Amigo never got into fights, but chasing balls was something I could not entirely control. A realistic goal for me was to continue to train him to bring back my own ball, while knowing that he would at times take the chance 'to help someone else out' who might have thrown a ball for a less interested chaser.

— What kind of puppy trainer do you want to be for your dog? What are the main qualities you would like her to see in you? How would you make sure that you get this message across?
— What are the areas where your dog needs patience, maybe more patience than other dogs you (unfairly) compare her with?
— Where do you think persistence has helped you to achieve the outcome you want with your dog? Where did you need to change your expectations?
— What would be an unrealistic goal to set for your fur baby?

Puppies and your thoughts and emotions have a lot in common. Puppy training and how you can live better with your thoughts and emotions have a lot in common too.

Puppies are cute and wild, all over the place and impossible to control with words. They can easily put themselves in danger, as they lack the ability to gain perspective and reflect on their action before trying something out. Commands, yelling, threats and violence will not lead to any improvement and definitely not to a relationship with your puppy where you look into each other's eyes and see love, care and connection.

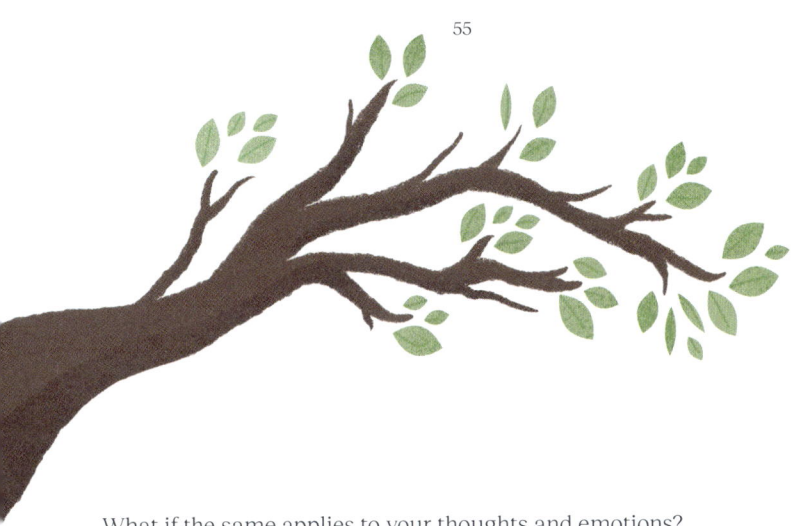

What if the same applies to your thoughts and emotions?

The main thing your thoughts have in common with puppies is that they just 'are'. Bouncing around, running in circles, tempting you to do whatever they come up with. Your emotions change course faster than Bailey, the greyhound, and they may be between collapse and hyperactivity, sometimes in the course of a few minutes. Emotions and thoughts are not your enemies. Like the energy and inquisitive mind of your puppy is not dangerous, bad or wrong, but thoughts and emotions can lead to unhelpful actions if they are not observed and guided, just like your puppy's overflowing energy.

And while you likely agree that puppies benefit from training, it is not equally acknowledged that your thoughts and emotions do too. Just to be clear. Thoughts and emotions are not trained to be different or to go away. You do not go to puppy training so your dogs have less energy and stop being curious about other dogs, life or bins. It is about training them to act in a way that it is not harmful for them or others. That is exactly the same goal set out here for you: to act in a way which is helpful for both you and others.

What if you could teach your observing self D.O.G. Relax (see page 40), the same way you taught your puppies so many different things?

What if you could really experience the fact that thoughts can't make you do something and that they are harmless mental events?

How much unnecessary suffering and pain could be prevented! How would you need to act as a trainer to encourage yourself to embrace D.O.G. Relax? What would this look like?

Let me assume that you asked around and someone recommended a puppy school. It is most likely that no one recommended a school with a harsh task master, who would scream at your canine companion and punish all failures. If anyone did, you would question how this could lead to success and a positive relationship between you and your dog. But a trainer described as patient, friendly and 'just great' would make you want to try them out.

Your inner mind observer, as I will call the position, needs the same qualities as a good puppy trainer:

— Patience
— Perseverance
— The ability to set realistic goals, regarding what you do (and not what you should think, believe, or try to forget).

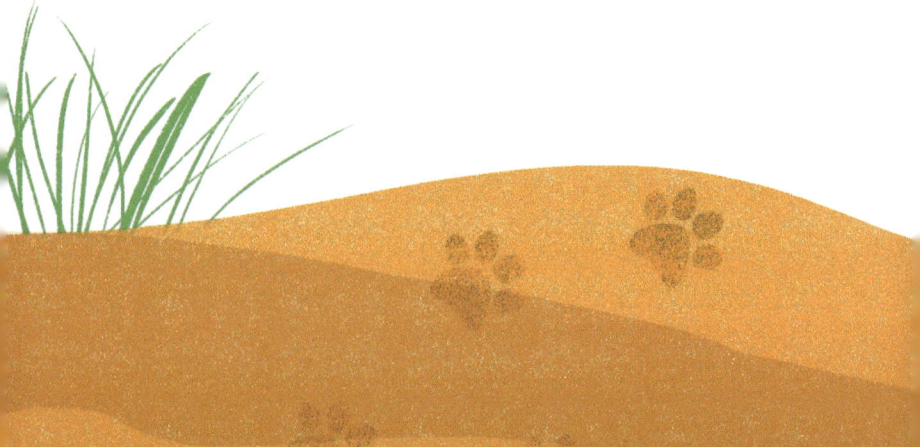

Let's say your cute little fur ball has found out where you leave your sneakers after coming home. Whether you call it an urge or just an internal drive for fun, the sneaker will be carried around and chewed, until there is not much left. If the little labrador is not trained to leave shoes alone (and kitchen sponges and socks), you would have to constantly replace these chewed items. Or maybe even take the poor dog to the vet to help her 'digest' the sponge she swallowed.

Without an inner mind observer, this is very similar to how you would run your life, with the highest priority being to satisfy your urges the moment they arise. It could mean shopping, eating, drinking or watching TV all night. This is not bad, but it is no fun for Frizzy if his owner is too lazy to go for a walk and Frankie would be disappointed if you were too tired to start a new day with her.

Nothing you do or don't do is 'bad', as there is also no such thing as a bad thought or a bad emotion. But too much of whatever you might be doing is stopping you from living the life you would like to live and could live instead. No thought or emotion can hold you back from doing what matters. So you do not need to fear them or invest in strategies to change or get rid of them. As always, the choice is yours, but a trained mind observer will help you to see that you have a choice.

Sometimes you will come across tempting offers, promising to help you buy better, eat less, stop drinking or start exercising - just like that. It sounds like a miracle, easy and full of promises.

In reality, it is hard work to change habits. Just as hard as it is for some labradors not to eat the kitchen sponge. And your inner mind trainer often uses methods you would never agree with in puppy school: criticising, blaming, punishing or giving up in anger or exhaustion.

Would your dog be there for you and as happy in his world as he is now if you had given up after he pulled on the leash or mistook your headphones for a toy? Patience and perseverance made a difference in his life and in the life you have together.

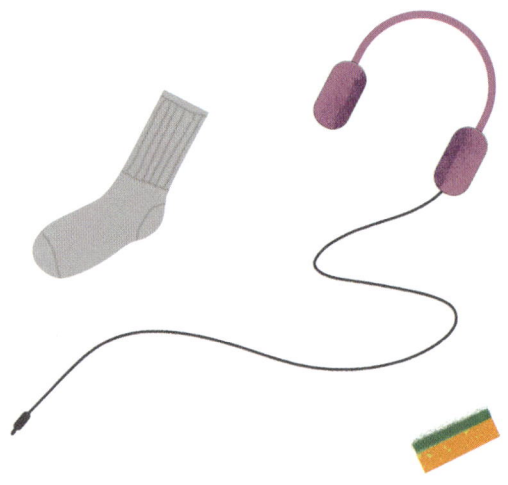

Patience and perseverance will make a difference to your thoughts and emotions and in your life. It won't always be comfortable, but you know from puppy school that following through with consistent actions is the best advice.

You set realistic goals for your dog by judging his potential and abilities after you got to know him. You can do the same by observing yourself. While we are all similar in many ways, we are all different in others. Expecting every dog to climb fences and fit in a small carry bag is as unhelpful as expecting every human to be good at ballet and weightlifting.

We all have a near endless number of thoughts, although we can only be aware of some at any given time. If that sounds strange, try it out. Say you are reading while you are sitting in a park. One of your thoughts right now is with the book and what you are reading. If I ask you to close your eyes at the same time, you would be able to tell me a few things about what just happened around you. Now that I have drawn your attention to your surroundings, your mind might wander away from the book and check out the trees, people or dogs.

Regardless of what you might have heard before, the most realistic goal for your mind is to stop trying to control your thoughts – but do try to notice them. You might wonder if that will lead to having crazy thoughts and doing more 'bad' stuff. That is a concern many people have, myself included, when I first heard about letting my thoughts just be and not challenging or trying to change them.

My words should not convince you, but practising and noticing can.

LISTEN TO YOUR THOUGHTS

Notice your thoughts and what you feel. Just notice and name them. You will need patience to listen. You will need the patience of a good dog trainer, so that you don't try to correct your thoughts and make yourself feel differently from how you feel right now. If this starts to be overwhelming, put your hand on your best four-legged friend and breathe out and slowly in. Feel your hand touching the soft fur and take your time.

Your thoughts and emotions might jump around like all those dogs in the dog park in the late afternoon, when owners finish work and it is finally playtime. They chase each other, get into a bit of a play fight, sort it out, move on, run fast, walk slowly, lie down or follow each other around.

Watch your thoughts like you watch these dogs. When you focus on one thought and get lost in it, notice that there are many others around it, like there are many other dogs in the park. Notice your thoughts and name them. 'Oh, here is the thought ... again.' Just like you notice the same black dog coming to the park every day at around the same time.

Some thoughts have become a story and you can choose a headline. Just like the giant poodle balancing on the retainer wall was named 'Queen' in my mind. It's not an exercise you can do once and then you are done. It is like teaching your dog to go outside for a wee and not to use the rug in the hallway. You needed to do it again and again.

With persistence and perseverance your little puppy was able to build new neural pathways, and when she felt like a wee she automatically went to the door to be let outside instead of going to the rug in the hallway. You helped her to notice and then to make a more helpful choice to maintain peace in your household.

Puppy's behaviour, like your thoughts and emotions, is not 'bad'. It is just what puppies do. However, some of the things puppies do are not helpful, like eating sponges, chewing runners or using the hallway rug as a toilet.

Please notice that I deliberately replace the words 'bad' or 'negative' with 'not helpful'. The world would be a different place if you could do this everywhere you went.

When you made choices on behalf of your puppy, you did so to help her to be safe, become a good companion and an enjoyable housemate. That is what you want your actions to achieve too.

Deep down, everyone wants to be safe, even though you might, at times, be tempted to metaphorically run off-leash across a road. Deep down you want to be loved and to love in return. Yet at times you disappoint others and yourself with unhelpful actions.

Let thoughts and emotions be. Label them as helpful or unhelpful regarding certain goals or situations, while getting to know them and their intentions. It can feel uncomfortable to stop the fight. With practice it will become easier and less challenging – just like it is for a dog who has learned not to pull on the leash, but to walk with it.

Take a thought for a walk

— What happens if you let thoughts just be, like you let the dogs
be in a dog park?
— What happens if you focus on one dog in the dog park only,
like being hooked by a thought?
— What happens if you take your focus from one specific dog to
others in the park, just like noticing that you are not only having
one thought, but many others at the same time?

 ## Overcome your inner schweinehund

This is a very challenging suggestion, but let me put it to you.
You have the choice to either overcome this inner schweinehund,
or to leave it for another time.

Remember that the best way to approach a challenge is with
puppy steps. A wobbly attempt in the desired direction with enough
praise and encouragement will lead to firmer steps towards what
is helpful for you and others.

— What would be an action you could choose, even if it creates
some discomfort, instead of doing what feels good for a moment
but leaves a bitter taste afterwards?
— Is there something sitting on your shelf needing attention
and you know it wouldn't feel good to address it?

Yes, it feels better right now to ignore the shelf and what is on it.
But tonight, the bitter taste will be that another day has passed
and you have not given time and energy to something that you
would like to have resolved.

An example from the world of humans might not fit. I've chosen to mind-read Tacco, a black and white Welsh corgi. Tacco has learned that if nature calls, he should stand in front of the terrace door to be let out. But he's lying in the hallway and having a snooze and feeling a certain urge, so he has the thought that it would be easier and quicker to just use the rug. It would be warm and comfortable.

Then he remembers that he has a choice and a chance to overcome his inner schweinehund, even if it means the discomfort of getting up and bracing the cold outside.

Because he loves the person who cares, feeds and grooms him, he chooses to do what helps this relationship to further grow and blossom. He gets up and walks to the terrace door.

Embracing discomfort led to him being called 'a good boy', patted and tickled behind his ear. It was worth doing what mattered and not following a thought with the invitation to avoid momentary discomfort.

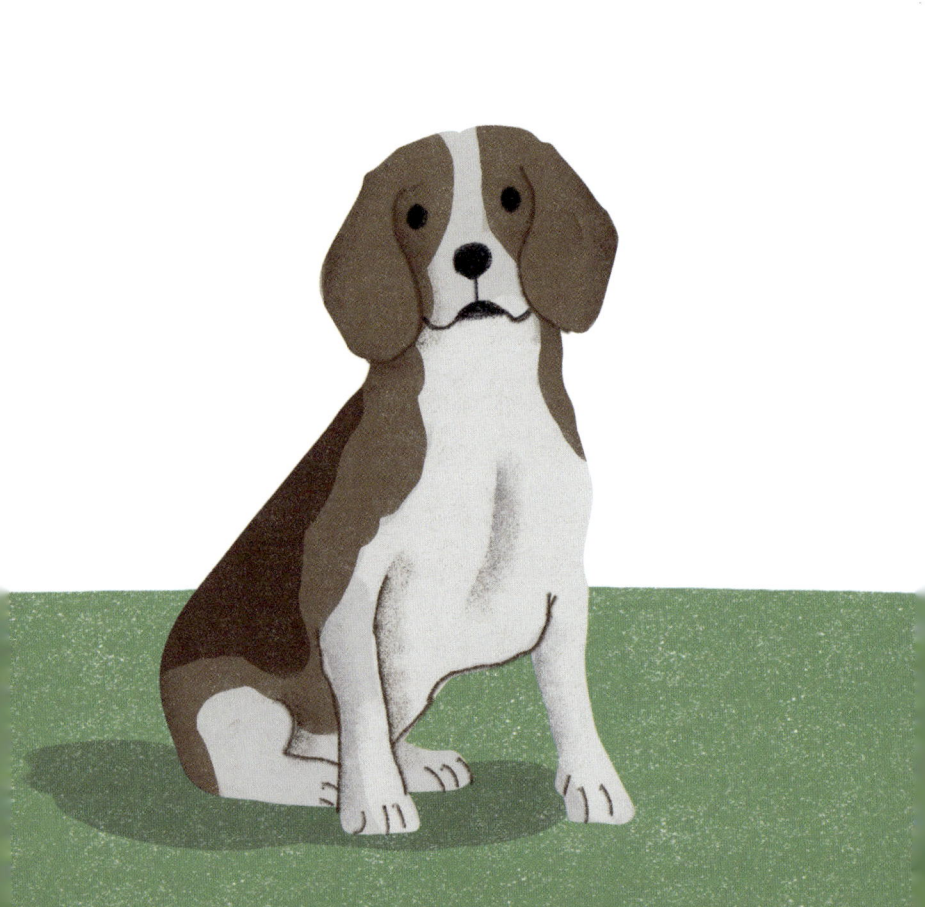

Go to your mat!

The world can only seem a safe place
when we feel safe inside.

Agapi Stassinopoulos

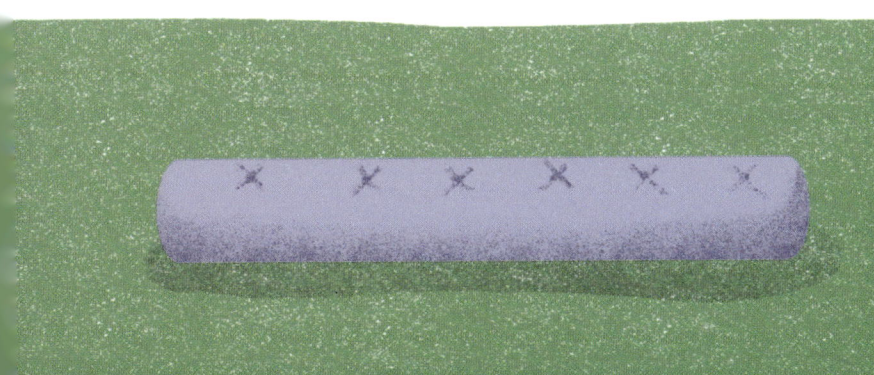

Most likely, and with lots of excitement, you went shopping or looking for a bed, cushion or mat for your new best friend to rest on before you brought her home. Young dogs need a lot of rest, and a sleeping puppy on a cosy, comfortable cushion on the floor is one of the best and nicest ways of getting respite from life's demands and challenges. Young dogs are often overcome by tiredness and will fall asleep wherever they were standing. If you notice that the little legs are moving more slowly and energy needs to be replenished, you might say, 'Go to your mat and have a rest'. I will use the word 'mat', even though it is probably much more than just a mat that you have prepared for your puppy to sleep on.

'Mat' is used in most dog training. It is, of course, much shorter than saying 'Go to your plush pink fluffy little princess corner'. However, there is no need to change whatever word you choose.

'Mat' is short, but does not beat the German command 'Platz', which is easily understood and liked by quite a few people who heard me talking to Amigo in German. Yes, he was bilingual, a genius. And yes, I am biased! I have to admit that I used German for commands I really meant and English as my 'love language'. But the command 'Platz', even sometimes voiced loudly, still came from a place of care, as I knew that being send to his mat was helping Amigo in many different ways.

What you have in common with your four-legged companion is that you want to feel safe. While dogs can sleep anywhere, they will only do so in a relaxed manner if they feel safe. Having a place to go to where he feels safe helps him to return to a calm state.

Most dogs get very excited when visitors arrive. They want to greet them, jump up and lick their faces. Some dogs grow tall and some visitors might not be strong, or they are scared of a dog so close to them. It is therefore helpful for a dog to learn to go to his mat, not to act on an impulse and to interact with a visitor when he is calmer.

Dogs, like humans, are social creatures, who love the company of others around them, unless they have been hurt and have lost trust in people and sometimes the world. Puppies are nearly always born with siblings and immediately form playful bonds. Young dogs love to follow their owners. If humans have hurt you and a part of you feels safer alone, you will love the company of your dog to make up for the people who are not in your life.

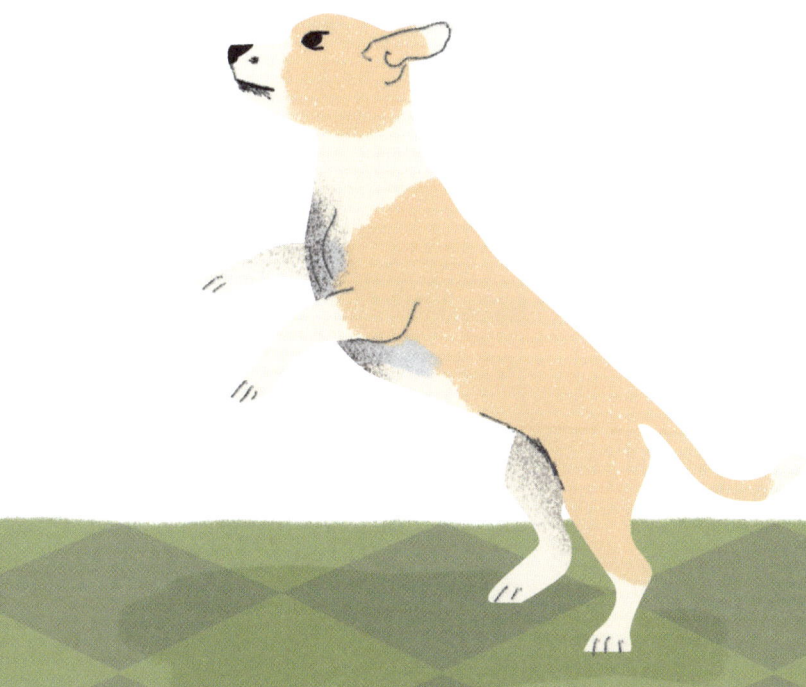

There are situations where the two of you cannot be together. You might have to go to a meeting, shopping or to see a doctor. What you can do before leaving home is to tell your dog that you will be back soon – something I never forgot to do. Yes, Molly will miss you immediately, maybe feeling the minutes like hours. However, having trained Molly to go to her mat and to calm down and feel safe will help her in this situation. She may even sleep the biggest chunk of the time while you are away.

The importance of a safe place to turn to was also invaluable for Smurf, who developed the habit of opening the cabinet door underneath the kitchen sink - easily done with click and release technology - to have a taste of the leftovers in the bin.

As you know, scolding a beagle for what beagles 'have to do' will not improve matters. Smurf is better sent to her mat and distracted with a chew toy, while her owner makes a promise to not leave leftovers so easily accessible.

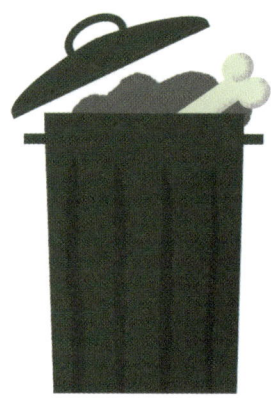

Smurf is visibly not happy, as she is led away from the most attractive bin. She is a bit agitated and tries to communicate that these treats are going to waste unnecessarily. Her owner encourages her to take her favourite chew toy, a chicken with a squeaky sound. Smurf chews on it vigorously and makes several attempts to sneak back to the kitchen. She is calmly, but firmly, sent back to her mat. Smurf has learned a lot and one thing she has learned is that her owner does not give up. While the first lessons were short and she got rewarded for one leg, two legs, three legs on the mat, the expectation is now that she will settle and stay.

And she does! Her chewing becomes less frantic, the chewing noise softer and, finally, with a big sigh, she puts her head down and dozes off. Watching a dog settle and then starting to breathe evenly and fall into a soft slumber is one of the best mindfulness exercises. I highly recommend it.

When training a dog, the mat should never be a place for punishment, as it makes it impossible to be a safe place as well. Even if your puppy needs a lot of encouragement and much petting, or verbal praise or little yummy treats, don't give up. Having a safe place will be beneficial for the rest of your dog's life.

Having a safe place to return to is important for humans too. You cannot always go to your 'mat' or fly away to an island and leave it all behind. So what can you do when you get agitated and are tempted to do what might not be beneficial? You are in danger of doing damage to yourself and others, even if you do not mean to, when you are triggered, see fight or flight as your only options, or when you are on autopilot and not making deliberate choices.

Go to your mat!

This is when you can feel lost, unsure and start blaming others, and ultimately yourself. You might at times like to give up on this whole difficult thing called life.

We are all in need of an inner 'mat' we can take with us, wherever we go. This 'mat' needs to be cosy, safe and help us to feel the feelings but not be overwhelmed by them. You need a 'mat' that reminds you that no feeling can be bigger than you are because it is you who is holding the feeling – and not the other way around. Keep this in mind.

You need a 'mat' you can turn to until you are ready to take the next step in line with how you truly want to be. You need a 'mat' where you can be with your pain, gently making room for it, to just be, until the waves get smaller and the storm will not blow you away.

I think it is worth reading the last paragraph again.

For many years, I had no idea that we can all carry our own 'mat'. And if we do, it will become easier to stay calm: not like a robot, but like a suffering human knowing that this feeling will change.

Holding on to this knowledge when waves are high and storms are howling is not easy. It was not easy for your puppy to go to his mat. Yet, when you look at him you know that it was helpful not to give up.

When you teach yourself to go to your inner peaceful place, take small puppy steps. Don't expect perfection. Making a start is a step towards a calmer inner future, regardless of what happens around you.

Create your 'mat' in exactly the same way you chose the mat and the position for it for your puppy; you wanted it to be as nice and as comfortable as it possibly could be for the new love in your life.

The following exercise will help you to create a peaceful place in your mind. It will be your own 'mat' that you can return to whenever you want to.

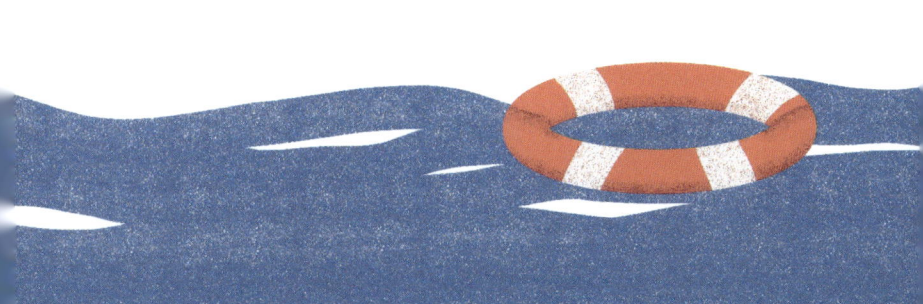

CREATING YOUR OWN 'MAT'

You can close your eyes or keep them open, softly focusing on your trusted companion resting on his mat or next to you on your couch or bed.

Imagine a place you have been to, or one you have seen in a movie, dreamt of or read about, and where you felt at peace.

While you go through your inner image and memory library, movies you have watched, places you have visited or documentaries you have seen, notice if you feel relaxed and comfortable. If not, wiggle and adjust, until it feels right.

Search a bit longer, and I am sure an image or a memory will come up.

Feel free to create a collage of different places in your mind.

When you find an image or a memory that seems just right, stay in that place and start to describe what you can see.

Do it so that you can truly see what you saw then, or do it to bring your collage together, with all the different elements you are imagining.

Is it inside or outside? Is the sun shining? Is it cloudy? Windy? What is the temperature like?

What can you hear? Are there any sounds or is it absolutely silent?

Take your time to feel your hands and your feet.

Can you touch anything?

What is the ground like?

Are you sitting, standing or lying down?

Relax your jaw and breathe, and notice the smells.

Move your tongue along the roof of your mouth and see if you can taste anything.

Stay there for as long as you want.

When you are ready, take a few deep breaths, let yourself know that you can always return to this place, stand up, roll back your shoulders and take a few steps.

You have just created your own 'mat', a peaceful place you can take with you no matter where you go and what is happening around you.

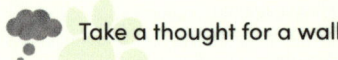

Take a thought for a walk

If you have done the exercise, think about how and if your emotions changed.

— Did you feel the same before, during and after you
   went back to your inner peaceful place?
— If something has changed, what and how?

Maybe it was your first time and you could only manage 'one foot on the mat'. Maybe you didn't attempt the exercise at all.

If so, take the following thought for a walk.

— What would have happened if you had given up so easily
   on your puppy or not even attempted to teach her to go
   to her mat or hop on your bed?
— How would she feel if there was no place in your home
   where it was safe for her to rest?

You can probably hardly bear this thought. So how can you deny yourself your own peaceful place?

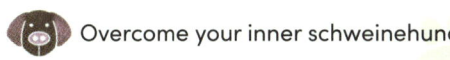 **Overcome your inner schweinehund**

It can be very challenging to be invited to go to a 'safe', peaceful place. You noticed the inverted commas? Exactly! How can you ever know or trust that a place is safe or truly peaceful? Maybe you wonder if there is anything like a peaceful place for you at all. This thought, like words or memories, can trigger your alarm centre, causing your body to get ready to help you to survive. Thank your brain for being on guard and make sure it is aware that you are here now and not in the past, when you might not have been safe.

Putting trust in me telling you that I know there is such a place inside you and that you can access it any time probably won't help. Because why would you choose to trust me? Many lived experiences of humans who know true deep pain look and feel like a huge and difficult inner schweinehund to overcome or live with. They seem too dangerous and threatening to even go one step closer.

But you have a trusted ally right by your side.

Join your best friend on her mat, put one hand on her side and try to imagine a place where you felt a little sense of peace. Stay there, and do not go towards what might happen next or what happened before. Right here and now, you are sitting with someone you trust, and the only place you go to in your mind is an image, one memory, which feels more peaceful than many others. Maybe it is just a short flashing image, like a little glimpse, and that is okay and might be enough for today. It is not a competition; it is not a must.
It is just an arms wide open invitation you can dare to follow.

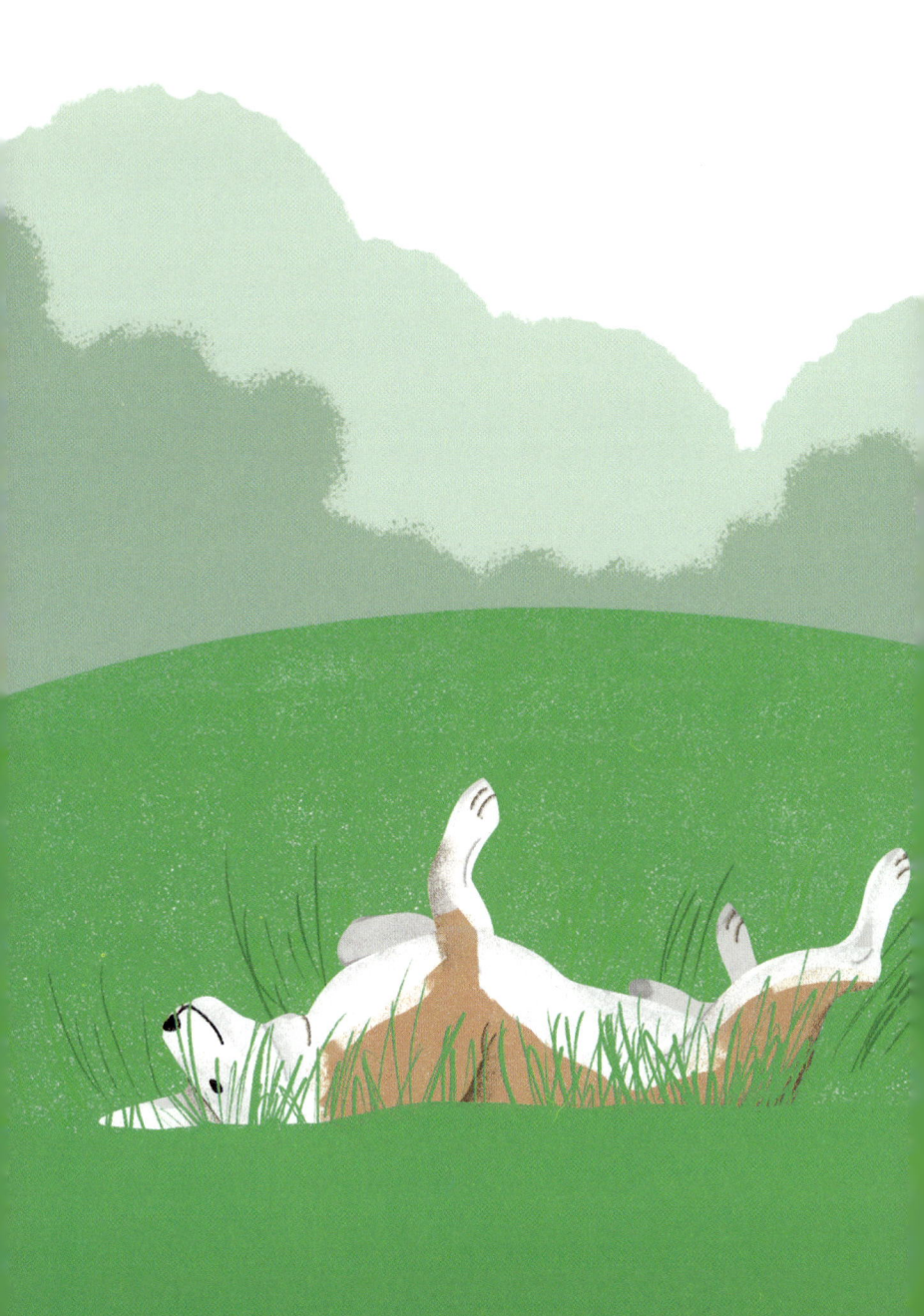

Why did you feed your dog today?

What matters most is to focus
on what matters most.

Roy T. Bennett

Adog always seems so motivated! Have you ever watched a dog starting its day? Getting up, slowly or quickly, depending on how she feels. Stretching, looking around and then just getting on with it. If they are healthy, most dogs are always up for a walk, a cuddle, some playtime, digging into their food and maybe begging for some extra little treats. When Amigo finally ran out of steam – and that took a long time – he went to his mat, circled on it a few times, lay down, let out a huge sigh, closed his eyes and fell asleep. It is not surprising that the life of a well-loved dog is often described as the best life and one to envy. A dog's life seems so effortless and full of energy. They never seem to lack direction or the motivation to engage in what's next.

It is unfortunate or fortunate, depending on how your day has been, that humans are different from their four-legged companions.

A dog's motivation is driven by what they like and want. Some dogs like to chase balls and they will. If not, they must like you enough to chase the ball and bring it back to you. If they like sniffing your pocket, they will walk alongside you without pulling the leash, hoping to be rewarded with a treat.

Dogs eat when they are hungry, and some eat more than they should, according to the scale and charts in the vet's office. And they continue to do so if we let them. Notice how similar we are to our dogs. However, there is a difference between a dog and its owner. You can look at charts and read about life expectancy and can then make choices in your dog's best interest. Even if their eyes are totally irresistible.

While making choices sounds like an attractive concept, it can create a dilemma too. Getting up in the morning is a joy for your four-legged friend, no doubt about it. A healthy dog would not spend a day on the mat, without an urge to move.

Most of us have experienced mornings when we have been tempted to just stay in bed. Nothing seems appealing enough to motivate you to get up and face the day. It might have been a day with a specific challenge or just a freezing cold morning. You might feel like nothing matters and that you have lost the spark you had a long time ago, or lost a love of life that you can see in a puppy bouncing around.

No human can be like a dog. But just as you make choices about your dog's diet, you can also make choices about your next step.

So when it all feels too hard, go slow. Don't push, don't debate. Don't call yourself names or describe yourself in a way you wouldn't talk to your old dog, even if she can't jump up with excitement like she did many years ago.

Go slow and use the voice you would use for Lady, who is now twelve and has some soreness in her joints and stiffness in her hips, especially when the mornings are cold.

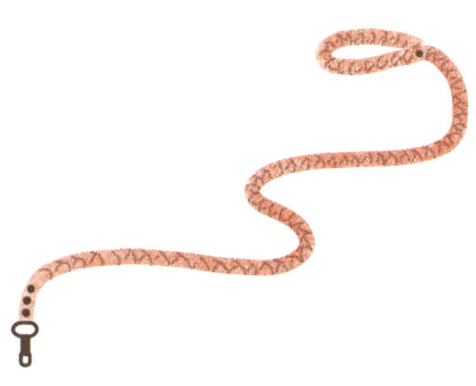

Why did you feed your dog today?

GO S.L.O.W.

STRETCH

Stretch one leg and then the other. Stretch out one arm and then the other. Round your spine. Make your dog your teacher and follow her lead.

LOOK

Look forward to one thing you enjoy. Even if you only enjoy it a tiny bit. If you can think of something that makes you smile, even better. A tiny thing can be to imagine stroking Goldie's soft flappy ears, just where the fur is like a mixture of velvet and silk.

or

Think of your Alfie, throwing himself on his back, offering his white and fluffy chest to be massaged, tickled and petted.

I am sure there is one very special thing you can think of and look forward to when thinking about your furry friend. Maybe you can even form a soft smile in anticipation.

This is what makes me smile, even now. Amigo could hear from afar that I had reached the bottom of a yoghurt tub with my spoon. He knew that his 'job' would be to lick the last little bit from the container walls and the bottom of the tub. If it was a larger one, his face would be inside, including his eyes, and he would hold the round plastic container with his paws and lick in circular motions.

He loved his 'job' and probably wondered why I stood there, watching and smiling and telling him what a very good and useful part of my household he was, and that his contribution to the recycling was invaluable.

OBSERVE

Observe your thoughts. What is your mind telling you? Just notice and let the thoughts come and go. Those thoughts are just mental events. They can't tell you what to do next. One might be about what you should/must/have to do – another might be about giving up.

All thoughts are already there, so do not waste your time trying to get rid of them. The secret to your dog's happiness and motivation is not being able to have all those complicated thoughts. A dog's motivation comes from what seems appealing and is in front of her.

Notice what happens when you are breathing and keep your attention in the present moment.

When you feel your body relax, your breathing is calm and your mind is clear, then it is time for the next step.

WISE

A wise decision is a decision you made when you were calm and deliberate. You know long afterwards why you made the decision. A wise mind can see your feelings, like not wanting to get up, and it can also see what truly matters to you. And so you can choose to face the rain and walk your dog.

Think about a choice you have right now. You can either continue to read this book, or you can ... . If you continue to read because you are too angry to respond to an email or too flat to hang the washing, it might be called a 'good choice' by some. Yet it is not a wise and deliberate choice, as your mind is not calm, clear and a helpful counsel.

If you went through this exercise – and one of your values is to show love for your dog by creating the fluffiest bed – putting the book down might be a wiser choice, rather than avoiding getting up. You can look back and find reasons why you can be proud of your action.

Right now, you have the choice to ... or to ... .

Ask yourself, what are both options based on? Feelings, emotions, thoughts, 'shoulds', 'musts' or values? What matters and what do you want to stand for as a person/dog parent?

A wise mind is a mind that stops at a crossroad and decides to go down the path called 'doing what matters'. A confused, clouded mind that is not fully aware of lots of worrying thoughts might choose to do what feels good or choose to avoid feeling at all. To access your wise mind takes calmness, courage and commitment.

Doing what matters and what is important to you in your heart, can feel incredibly nice, fluffy and right. Recall the day when you got your puppy and you fed her for the first time? I remember cooking a small portion of rice and mixing some minced meat in it. I stood there with a warm feeling and just watched Amigo having his first meal at my place.

Of course, in the following years, there were countless mealtimes, and the memory of how I felt during the first meal faded. Feeding became part of a routine. It brought some inconvenience, like buying dog food and carrying it inside. Once I bought the wrong food and had to find someone who would take it, which also meant going out again and getting the correct one so Amigo's stomach was not further upset. He also got used to being fed at a certain time, so coming home started with the priority of feeding Amigo and not having a cup of tea and a biscuit, which I would have preferred at times.

Why did I and all of you reading this book continue to feed our dogs? Why do you walk her in sun, rain or snow? Why is there no question that you will take her to the vet when sick, even if she might throw up in the car or wake you up during the night?

You do it because when you come to the crossroad, consciously or not, you choose to go down the path of doing what matters. Some of you might think that you do not have to make a choice about feeding your dog. You might think that this is just what a dog owner does, or needs to do, but you do it because it matters to you that your puppy rolls on the grass with a full stomach. However, what truly matters is not always so obvious and so relatively easy to do.

I want to go back to the example of deciding whether to get up or stay in bed. Your brain debates to and fro between getting up, something you should/must/have to do, or staying in bed, something you would like to/feel like/want to do.

How can we make a choice that comes from a wise mind?

We need to identify what truly matters to us. We need to get to know what is most important to us or, in other words, what values we want to pursue.

It is worth stopping here for a moment and clarifying what values are. Values are often described in terms of what someone wants or their goals. A dog lover might say, 'I value having a house with a backyard for my dog'.

Here, having a house with a backyard is not a value but a goal. It can be ticked off when achieved. A value is something you pursue knowing that you can never tick off a list. Choosing your values means choosing the way you want to be.

And while having a house with a backyard is or might be a goal worth chasing, the value of love and care and having fun with your four-legged bundle of energy can be lived today in the park or in the smallest apartment.

For a deeper dive into values and how they are different from goals, check out *The Happiness Trap*, listed in the resources on page 172.

So Lady is taken to the park, even when it rains, because what truly matters is to live the values of love, care and fun. Even if it does not feel good, even if there might be thoughts about not wanting to leave the bed or the house, and even if coming home leaves a trail of dirt from the front door to the bedroom.

On days where you feel that you haven't done anything and when it all seems too hard, remember that you did feed your dog, and so you did something based on what truly matters to you.

Happiness can be a fleeting moment when all stars seemingly align, like the puppy's first meal in your house. But the deeper happiness of purpose and meaning is encountered when you face your pain, fear and doubts, and do what you know is truly important to you anyway. When you do what counts and become how you want to be, regardless of whether only your four-legged best friend is watching, then you can go to bed knowing that you did your best.

Do dogs follow values too? There are documentaries and YouTube videos of animals helping others in a seemingly selfless way. Some argue that this is part of their instinct and not a deliberate choice, which does not answer the question of 'Why?'. Some argue that dogs clearly do have values, others say that not enough is known to make a final judgment. What is known from observation is that dogs don't sit for hours pondering one thought before, for example, deciding to go for a swim.

I have simplified the reason why animals help others in my own mind. I think that they do so because all living beings know that it is better for us, our neighbours, our community and the world if we support and help each other. This can be called a value.

However, dogs do make mistakes too. They can make choices which are unwise that do not contribute to peace and harmony. There's more about this in the next chapter.

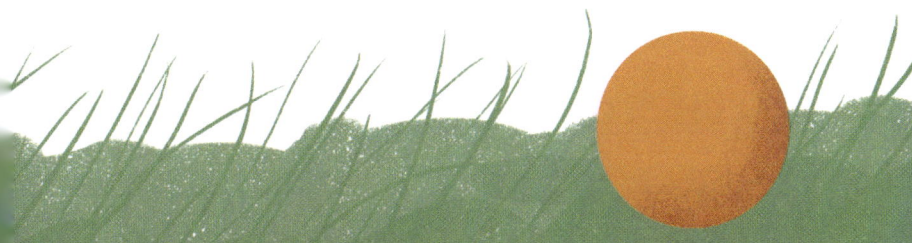

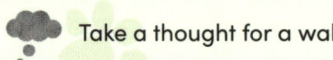 **Take a thought for a walk**

We go on many walks with our dogs. Shorter walks just to the next nature strip, or much longer walks to the park or along a river or a beach. Pick one or two questions that stand out to you, and take them on a shorter or a longer walk.

— What is one thing that matters to you today?
— What could you do to walk one step on the path of doing what matters, either for your dog or for yourself? (Is there paperwork to be done, an email to be sent, a phone call to be made?)
— What is important to you in regard to your own health? And what would your dog see when you take action in that direction?
— What do you want to stand for? And what would it look like if you turned those values into actions?

You can come back to the other thoughts or questions and take them with you on your future walks.

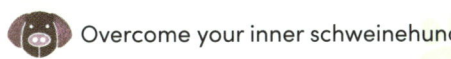 Overcome your inner schweinehund

It is easy to do what matters if it feels good. It is much more difficult and, at times, next to impossible, to do what matters when something feels scary, too hard or seemingly beyond your capacity to tolerate the pain and discomfort it might bring.

I recently saw a short video on Facebook showing a dog chewing his bone while two magpies cheekily pecked on his back and side flanks. The dog turned around a few times, but magpies are not scared off easily, and so the pair just continued to pick the dog's fluffy fur. I am not sure if they hoped that the dog would leave and donate the bone to them or if they were after a little piece of fluff to take to their nest. It looked relentless, and the dog clearly felt a sense of discomfort, having these two pecking at him, but he continued to chew on his bone. The saying, 'Like a dog with a bone' came to my mind. To him, the bone mattered more than paying attention to the two birds with their sharp beaks.

— What is your bone? And how do you decide to proceed when you want to hold on to it while you're getting pecked at?
— Do you give up the bone and let them have it? Do you talk yourself into not liking bones anyway?
— Or do you decide to hold on to your bone and continue to do what truly makes your heart sing, while noticing the pain of being pecked at and not giving up?

I know that many pains seem so much more unbearable than the pecking of two magpies. And yet, if you keep choosing the path of doing what matters, the pain will be outweighed by finding purpose and meaning.

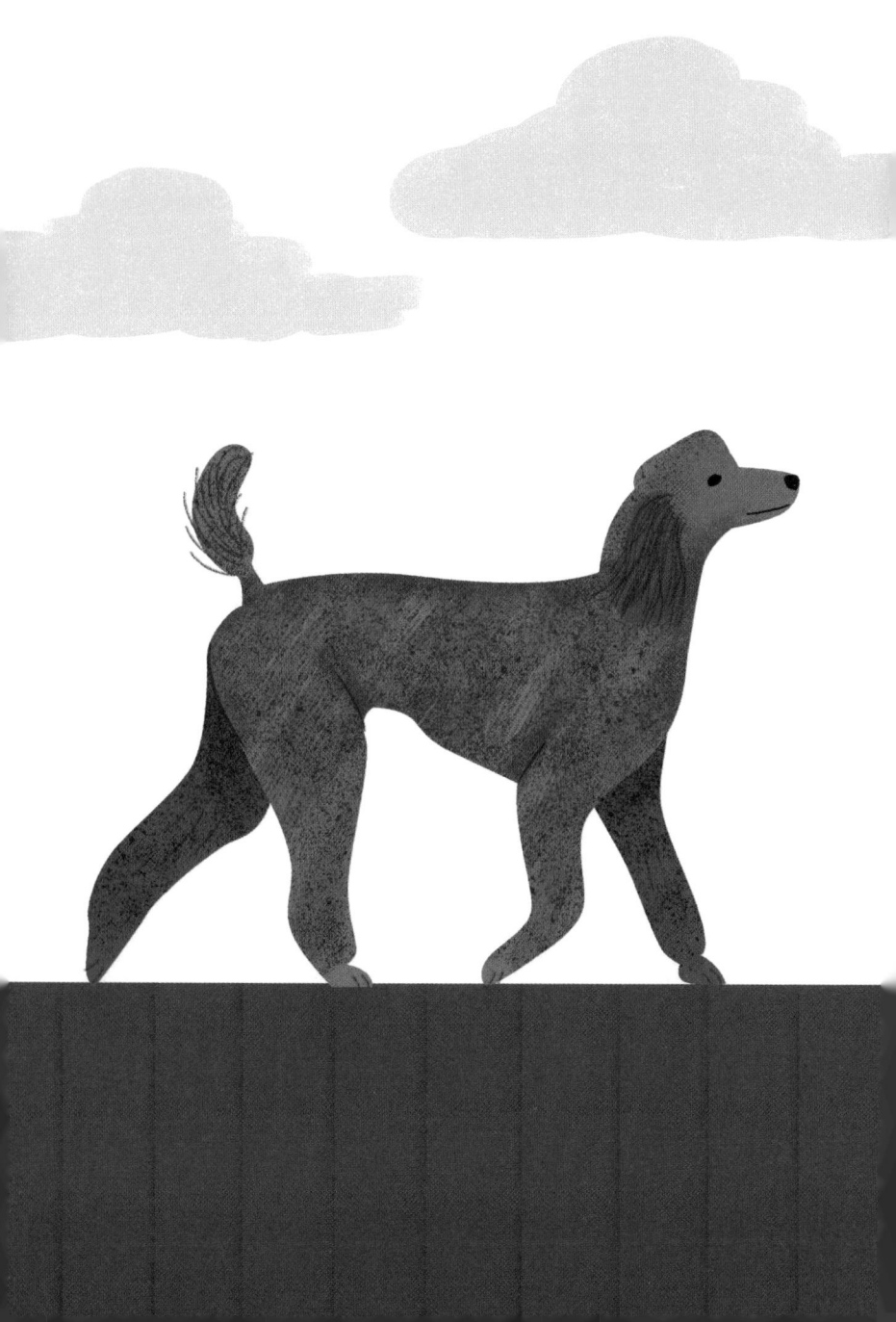

The cheesecake is gone!

Pleasure is the beginning and the end
of living happily.

Epicurus

The more importance we place on avoiding
unpleasant feelings in life, the more
our life tends to go downhill.

Russ Harris

The first quote calls us to avoid everything challenging or anything uncomfortable and that seeking pleasure is the recipe to having a great life. Avoiding discomfort is very human. You do not touch a hot stove because you know how long a burn can hurt, and you avoid it without really thinking about it. If you feel physical pain, you might take a painkiller. If your whole body aches with a body-mind pain and suffers from the difficulties of the world, you might try to avoid the world or do whatever it takes not to feel this kind of pain. The second quote points out the consequences of avoidance and that pleasure might be short-lived and lead to a life lacking meaning, connection and growth.

Do you agree with the first or the second quote? Come back after reading this chapter and notice if your view has changed or not. Our four-legged companions are not so different from us humans in their attempt to avoid what they dislike and in seeking pleasure.

I have been amused many times by a giant poodle being walked on a footpath next to a sandy beach. Dividing the footpath and the beach is a timber wall about forty centimetres high and fifteen centimetres wide. I do not know the name of the giant poodle, but she looks, behaves and walks like a queen. Head high, one leg in front of the other and not interested at all in sniffing the bottoms of other dogs passing.

Her owner - perhaps better described as her butler - tries to gently encourage the Queen to hop over the wall and enjoy some playtime with other four-legged friends on the beach, but the Queen decides

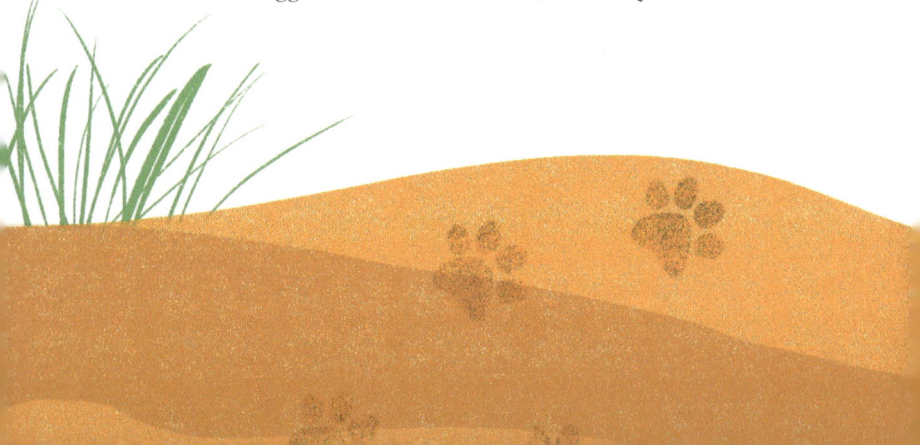

to use the barrier as a balance beam, and to look down on people on the footpath and at the dogs playing on the beach. No encouragement could ever make her step on sand.

When the Queen decides to balance on top of the retainer wall, she does so for a very good reason. Nothing dogs do is for no reason. We might not understand it, but there will be a purpose in everything they do. That is the same for us. Nothing you do is for no reason.

You don't know about everything going on in your dog's mind, even if you know her well. People will never know everything going on in your mind either, and you will never know everything about yourself. For example, something that might have happened to you a very long time ago that left an imprint on your body and soul.

Watching the Queen and her acrobatic avoidance to step on the sand, it became clear that she must have very good reasons for not walking on the beach. Maybe she once stepped on the sand and burnt her little paws. Sand can be very hot during summer in Melbourne. Or maybe there was another dog playing rough and it scared her. Maybe she wandered off mindlessly, as young puppies do, and had trouble finding her human protector in the shrubs near the beach.

I don't know the reason, but there will be one. Remember, nothing a dog does is for no reason. It must have made her feel uncomfortable in the past, or she was just not willing to give up her elevated position. I've even seen her turn around on it in an acrobatic act, preferring this to stepping down on one side or the other. True story!

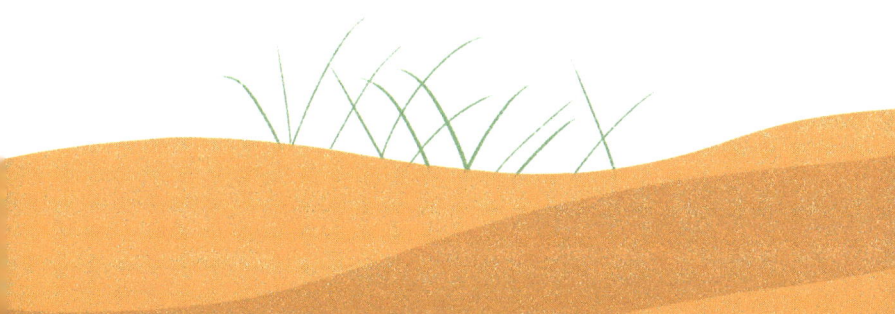

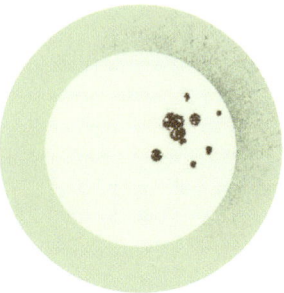

What the Queen missed out on was rolling in the sand, chasing other dogs to the water's edge or catching all kinds of flying objects thrown from other dogs' two-legged companions. A change in her routine would have required a degree of discomfort. Deciding something new or different will often make you and your dog feel uncomfortable. Change might feel difficult, but without a willingness to be uncomfortable some changes are impossible, your life will be less fun and you will not live the way you could if you dared.

The Queen was allowed to stick with her routine. But what if your dog's way of doing what feels good is not good for her or unacceptable to you?

Amigo's urge led him to do something that nearly made me cry. To understand this, you would have to be me, a German with a special love for cheesecake.

I grew up in Germany and moved to Australia when I was nearly forty years old. Many things are different here. I like to explore new places, enjoy all kinds of food and embrace the traditions brought to Australia by people from all over the world. There is a lot to love! However, one thing I cannot love, not even like, are cheesecakes made with cream cheese. A German-baked cheesecake, made of quark, which is very cheap and available in all supermarkets where I grew up, was one of the weekend treats, either at my place or when visiting someone around 3 pm in the afternoon.

Living here, I missed it. To find quark is a challenge and to pay for it a shock. But every now and then, I treated myself and made one according to an old recipe. One day, I took it out of the oven and put it on a rack on the kitchen bench to cool down. Knowing that the smell had called Amigo into the kitchen, I pushed the cake into the middle of the bench, so as not to tempt his nose any further. It was a cold and wet day, and I left Amigo inside during my short trip to the post office without thinking twice. I know, I shouldn't have …

When I came back there was no black fur ball greeting me with a wagging tail at the front door. I called him as this was very unusual. He walked slowly down the hallway with his tail between his legs, and I was sure that he was sick, so I touched his nose and of course asked him what was wrong. I was concerned.

And then I walked into the kitchen. All that was left on the kitchen bench was a clean plate with no trace of the cake. What I know now and didn't know then is that a kelpie cross can eat a cheesecake without suffering from an upset stomach. I was the one who was upset. Very much so. And his body language told me that he had a bad conscience as well. I will never know if he was in two minds before digging in, but from then on, Amigo had to suffer smelling the cheesecake in the oven and then see it being taken away to a place where he could not reach it. Being a dog and having dog-like limits and unique urges, it was clear to me that he would never be able to make wise choices around cheesecakes.

The cheesecake is gone!

He also had another rather unusual favourite food – tomatoes!

I had planted some tomatoes in pots on the sunny side of the house, but when it was almost time to enjoy my little harvest, nearly all the tomatoes had disappeared. I blamed the possums and told Amigo many times to make sure that they did not come near the plants. However, Amigo was far too peaceful to mind any intruder, and, as it turned out, I was blaming the wrong culprit. One day I saw him gently stripping ripe tomatoes off the plant and enjoying the juicy treat. It was too funny to interrupt him, and I just watched with a smile on my face. The coming year I was rewarded with lots of little tomato plants growing in all different areas of the garden.

Why Amigo jumped on the kitchen bench is easy to explain. He did what he thought was best for him in that moment. I do not think that he considered it as an act of kindness to help me avoid some extra calories. He missed the moment when he could have stopped and made a different choice.

Of course, that is beyond the ability of a beloved family pet who didn't go through intensive training.

Some of you would still prefer the New York-style cheesecake and never warm to the German one, even if I could present you with a freshly baked piece. And that is absolutely fine! We all have different likes and dislikes.

Which kind of cheesecake you prefer will not stand in the way of finding happiness, purpose or meaning in your life. However, following your nose and doing what might feel good for a moment might not always be the wisest choice either.

Rex is a German shepherd. He is vigilant by nature, loves to guard the house and garden and is fiercely loyal to his two-legged companion. He made life so much more bearable for his best friend during the COVID-related lockdowns. The not so frequent occasions when a visitor would step over the front door changed to no visitors at all. Walks were undertaken keeping the recommended safe distance, and the neighbour's cat kept a safe distance too, without needing a special recommendation.

Life in isolation suited Rex just fine. That this was not the best for everyone became apparent after the lockdowns had ended and an electrician was needed to fix a faulty light switch. It wasn't easy to get one for such a small task. When the tradesperson finally came to the house, Rex was beside himself. Instead of greeting the stranger, he behaved in a way that was scary for both humans present. The owner was confused and apologetic and promised to put Rex in another room.

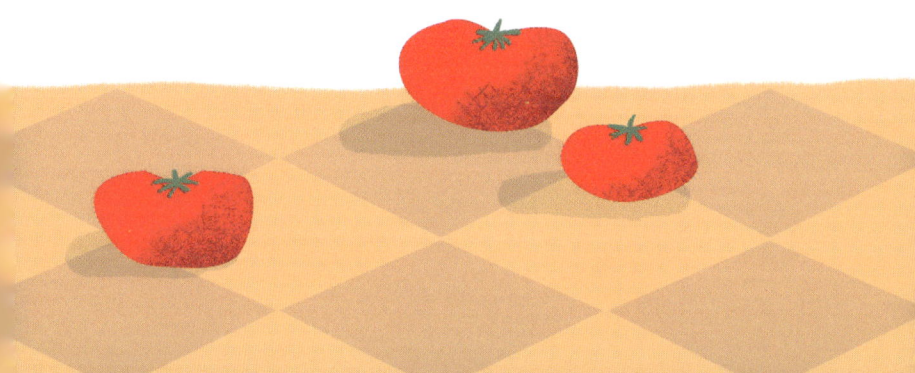

The electrician, who had already had a painful experience with
a customer's dog before, refused to enter the house and left. As a
consequence, the bathroom light did not get fixed.

Letting Rex continue to do what he did during lockdown would have
extended lockdown indefinitely and led to an isolated existence for Rex
and his owner. Rex and his most important person could not resolve this
issue without outside help.

A good dog trainer with experience and patience found the key and
the solution. Rex did what he thought was best in a situation where
he felt his best friend's safety was at risk. He made a judgement once
during lockdown that visitors were obviously not welcome in the house.
Rex had to learn to trust his owner's judgment more than his own.
Looking at his owner's face would tell him if this person had permission
to enter or if he would be rewarded for scaring them off. It did not
happen overnight and Rex erred on the side of caution. But he also
realised that visitors with a human permit to come in sometimes played
tug of war with him in the backyard or brought him a bone.

Being a protective watchdog, nobody could or should have entered the
house when Rex was the only one in command. Rex was right -
a stranger can be a danger. But he was not always right. Strangers can
become friends, play and be fun, and bring an unexpected treat!

As you will have noticed, this is not an easy chapter. We all want to
chase what we like and avoid what we don't. And that is both a human
and a dog's nature.

So what makes some people decide that they are better off experiencing discomfort, facing a challenge and doing what they have feared for so long? It is because otherwise they miss out like Queen, who will never chase a ball with other dogs along the beach, jump quickly into the waves and roll with pleasure in the sand.

It is because they know that when Amigo followed his nose and indulged himself he had a moment of pleasure, but an afternoon of regret.

It is because they understand that Rex's human housemate is happier with light in the bathroom and some visitors from time to time. Even if it means investing in a dog trainer and staying firm; and they can imagine that Rex is happier too.

Humans can decide to do what matters, even if it is hard, knowing that acting on an instinct or a reflex will not lead to a better life.

— What is one step you could consider - or do - which might feel like hot sand but leads towards something you have missed out on for so long?
— What could you do instead of following the seductive smell and overindulging? What could help you to not chase short-lived pleasure and suffer long term regrets?
— Is the price you pay for your safety strategies a good deal?
— What is one step you could take into the unknown, and who could be your trainer to help you with this? Maybe your trainer has four legs, or maybe two?

This was a challenging chapter and you might like to go back to your 'inner mat', a safe place you have hopefully created (see page 72).

Now we will walk down memory lane and I will invite you to remember the sweetness of the first touch.

The cheesecake is gone!

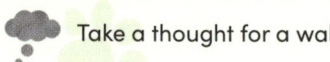

Take a thought for a walk

In your mind, take Queen the giant poodle for a walk. Imagine being her but with your own life story.

— What is the sand you fear?
— What do you do to avoid stepping on it, and what kind of balancing is required to stay on the wall and not step down?
— What is it you are avoiding at all cost?
— What is it you might miss out on?

In your mind be Amigo, left alone at home with an open door to the kitchen.

— What is a scent in your nose you follow at times?
— What can lead you to do something you regret the day after?
— What do you do without considering if the consequences are worth the moment of pleasure?

Before you read further, wait a moment. There are a lot of thoughts to take for a walk in the questions above. Do what the dog trainer did when working with Rex.

She went slowly, gently and with a lot of patience. Rex had felt his safety threatened, so pushing, coercing, coaxing or arguing with him to change his behaviour would just have threatened him more.

However, the trainer did work towards changing his way of jumping to conclusions, but gently, with love and kindness.

Please only continue with the following thoughts if you can be gentle with yourself, like the trainer was with Rex. Otherwise, it might trigger memories of feeling unsafe along with the urge to self-protect.

And as you are, of course, not Rex, you will not run to the door barking and scaring strangers away. But you might shut the book, feel like rolling up in a ball under the doona and give up.

You might keep the door shut to new experiences and maybe also humans who can become friends.

If any kind of feeling seems overwhelming, stop here and breathe, pat your dog and let her know that she is safe with you, and know that right now you are safe with her too.

 ## Overcome your inner schweinehund

When you are up for a challenge, consider the following:
— How do you try to keep yourself safe?
— What is the hurt or pain you try to avoid?
— What is one step you could consider – or do – that might feel like hot sand but could lead towards something you have missed out on for so long?
— What could you do instead of following your nose?
— What could lead to more helpful consequences?
— Is the price you pay for safety strategies a good deal?
— Where and how have you learned to react the way you react now?
— Is what you always did still leading you to the desired outcome when you consider the whole situation calmly, with courage and an awareness that you are an adult with choices?

In the past, what might have been a situation where you didn't have a choice is different here and now, even if it feels the same. Rex had to learn what is sometimes helpful is not always helpful. To consider different contexts and to be aware of the differences between then and there and here and now will be helpful for you too.

The cheesecake is gone!

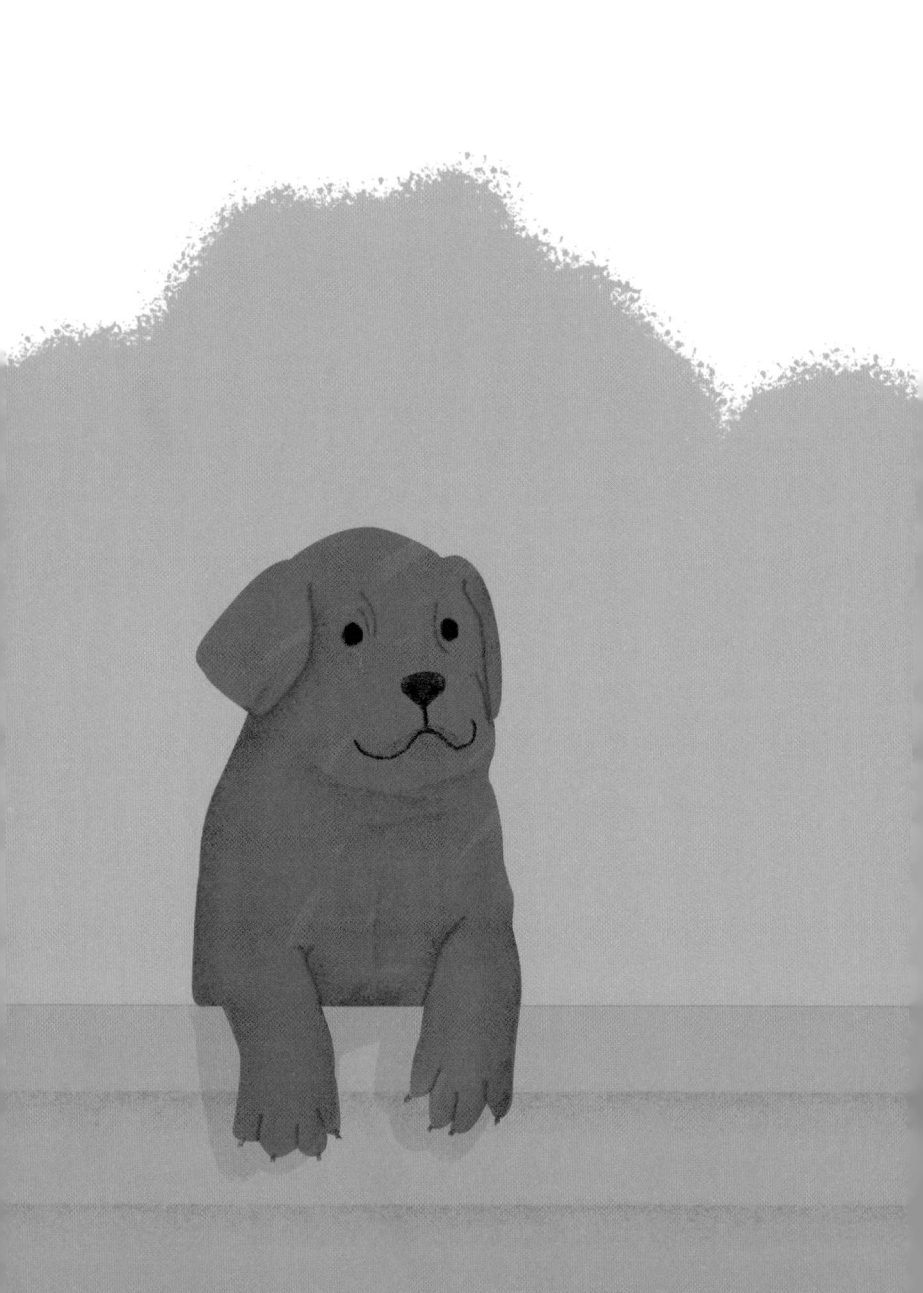

Holding your puppy for the first time

Little darling getting into my meditation
this morning, Namaste and all.
This puppy needs cuddles and breakfast.

Jo Stanley

It is a very special moment and one we all remember – the first time you held your puppy.

Think about when you took her home and couldn't take your eyes off her. Or maybe you adopted an older dog, who had already had many experiences before meeting you. It was still most likely love at first sight, and she became your baby, regardless of age and size.

In that moment, your heart opened and you felt happiness. But not only happiness. There was also the feeling of care, deep love and the start of a unique connection with this creature who would, you hoped, be around for many years to come.

Each first encounter is different and going back in your mind to this moment can feel a little bit like being there again. Your heart feels full, your arms want nothing more than to hold your dog and your hands only desire to stroke the soft fur. And when these cute eyes meet yours, an eternal bond is created. Your voice is soft and you tell her that she is beautiful, and will be loved and cared for. You promise that while it might be scary to be taken away from her siblings, or previous home, you will be her protector and help her to grow, have fun and be happy.

My life with Amigo started like this. Amigo was left at the Lost Dog's Home, weened too early from his mother.

When I held him for the first time, I promised him that his life would be better. Much better than his weeks inside a cage with all these barking dogs around. It was love at first sight, no doubt about it. And after the staff saw how quickly and deeply I fell for this little fellow, they told me what was 'wrong' with him. He had ringworm, which needed urgent treatment, his tail had been broken, which would make it bend at an awkward angle, and they were not sure what other neglect and mistreatment he might have experienced.

I had no intention of reconsidering my decision. He was already mine and mine to care for. Without doubt, I signed the paperwork and committed to being with his suffering - not knowing if it could be eased - to show him in any way I could that I truly cared. His past trauma and his current suffering opened my heart to love, care and showing him kindness, and to calming his anxiously beating heart. I knew that whatever happened to him, he would carry experiences and memories somewhere inside in ways I could never fully know.

Attending to his physical issues was not difficult at all. To get rid of ringworm is a straightforward matter. The name of the disease is very misleading. There are no 'worms' involved. It is a fungus that creates a round bald patch, which is treated with a combination of a topical therapy cream and an anti-fungus medication to swallow.

He didn't mind the cream, in fact he enjoyed the attention and rolled on his back the moment I approached with the tube in hand. Getting him to swallow the tablets took more convincing and some tricks.

The crooked tail grew curved sideways. When we love, we do not focus on the imperfect parts. We know that they are a part of every living creature and acknowledge the pain that was caused. We see the whole being, with a unique history, worthy of being loved and cared for.

At least, that's what we do with our dogs. We spend much less time doing this with ourselves. Unfortunately, we often do not make room for our own flaws and do not embrace ourselves with the same unconditional love.

Amigo was a charming, strong and clever dog who had survived against some odds. If I ever noticed his bent tail, I only took it as a reminder of what happened to him, which was totally unfair and of course not his fault. He could not have escaped, which is what he did from a fenced backyard at times as an adult. He could not have fought back. He never did that in his life. He was a loved and perfect companion.

Neither Amigo nor I could ever forget that he had been locked up under terrifying circumstances. Loving someone's - or our own - hurt parts does not mean to forget how they were created and by whom. It means to live with them with kindness and care.

Training Amigo was easy. Most of the time, he was quick to learn and eager to please. Yes, sometimes he was too eager to please other people by chasing the ball they threw for their dog. Nobody and no doggy is perfect. And of course, I still remember who ate the cheesecake ...

However, the terror he survived was suddenly evident in an everyday situation. After he had all his vaccinations, I decided to take him on a drive to the beach for the first time.

Usually playful and jumping he refused to hop into the back of the car. Not the softest blanket or a treat could make him get in. As he was still so little, I picked him up, explained to him what was going to happen, lifted him in and sat him on the blanket. All he could do was jump back out of the car. I tried again and again. Finally, I managed to close the back hatch. Before even leaving the garage, he started to climb to the front. The panic in his eyes and his movements were palpable.

No way would I restrain him or force him to stay there. His body must have remembered what happened to him, and it dawned on me that, of course, he was willing to do anything to avoid going through this trauma again.

How could his body ever forget the darkness and the too tight boot of the car that brought him to the Lost Dog's Home. He climbed over the backseat, squeezed between the two front seats and rolled into a ball in the foot space of the passenger seat. And that's where he travelled from then on. He never climbed up on the seat and never tried to sit on my lap. He was just happy and content that I 'got him'. To really understand his pain meant to take it seriously. I needed to be with him and not turn away.

I felt compassion for Amigo, not because I have ever been locked in a boot, but because I, like every being, know about suffering and pain.

I can feel deeply connected, loving and caring, even in moments when I do not know how to ease the pain or am unable to rewrite the story of its creation. Not all suffering can be eased in the foot space of the passenger seat.

My concern for the experience of pain, and paying attention to visible and invisible suffering is a choice. Pain and suffering is what connects all creatures. If you understand this in your heart, you will judge less and ask more: What happened to you? And what happened to me?

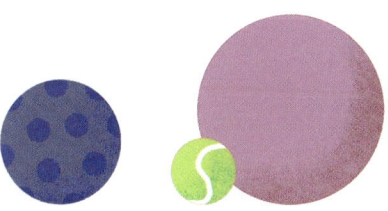

Holding your puppy for the first time

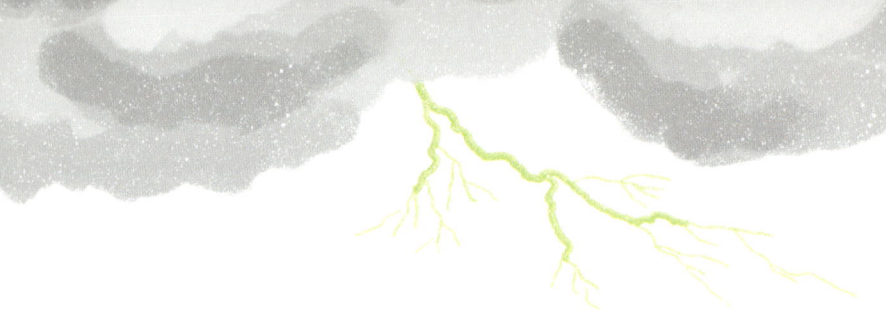

We need to listen to the memories stored in the body. Listening is more important than knowing the truth. All that has been is still present and can be triggered. The pain when being triggered is real. And the pain is what needs attention, love and care, not the details of a story. You might like to take a moment to let this sink in.

When memories get triggered, compassion is the only helpful response. Even if others judge, punish and might minimise the huge impact of what was done to you or your rescue dogs. When triggered, damage can be done. It was not Amigo's fault and is not the fault of any other survivor; it is what happens as a result of the unbearable pain of unhealed wounds.

Amigo got triggered in closed spaces and seemed to unleash what some would call a wild beast caged inside the most peaceful dog. At least, that is what it looked like and how it could be judged. Actually, it was the frightened little dog trying to do what he had done before. He tried to defend his right to be free and feel safe.

Many years later, I left Amigo for a few days with a dog-sitter at my place. I had told her that he was afraid of thunderstorms, friendly with the neighbour's chickens if one jumped the fence and that he avoided cats because he was afraid of them. We had this chat while watching Amigo playing with his favourite toy, a squeaking pig. I then told her about his feeding habits and made sure that she knew that he could not be locked up in any room. If inside the house, he needed to be able to walk around. He was also happy outside, but not at night and not during thunderstorms.

Unfortunately, when I came home, the timber frame of the bathroom door was destroyed as high as the poor dog could reach. The dog-sitter had locked him in while meeting a friend for dinner, and he had tried to chew his way out. The door was full of scratch marks from his attempt to break free. That would be costly to repair, but no money could repair the trust I lost in the dog-sitter. She, who had glowing reviews and said how much she loved and understood dogs, had not believed me and didn't notice that Amigo must have been clearly distressed when she locked him in the bathroom.

What she had done, of course not deliberately, still pains me. Most of you reading this, will take Amigo's side and feel his anguish, desperation and pain. These feelings show that you do care for a suffering creature, deserving love and care, as we all do. And you notice that you care, even knowing that Amigo has done damage that needed expensive, professional repair.

His suffering during this night might remind you of your own experiences when you were not listened to, let down and triggered. Take a moment to notice what is showing up. Put the book down and let your hand feel your beating heart.

Let yourself and your fur baby know that you are safe and loved, regardless of what has happened in the past. Let your dog know that you love them despite what they did when they got triggered. Let yourself know that you deserve love, regardless of what you did when you were triggered.

Take a thought for a walk

— How did you feel holding your puppy for the first time?
— Can you visualise the moment you got him in your arms?
— What were your thoughts?
— What would you say to your dog when they are afraid?
— What do you say to your dog when something gets damaged out of fear or panic?
— Would you ever punish a dog who is in pain, even if he caused damage you have to pay for?

Maybe the last question sounds ridiculous. If so, you are ready to tackle a challenge.

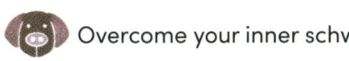 **Overcome your inner schweinehund**

— What if, when fear fills your heart and mind, you talk to yourself
in the way you would have talked to Amigo the night he was
locked in the bathroom?

— What if, when pain becomes a heavy stone in your stomach, you
breathe into it, you make room and hold the pain, like you held
your puppy for the very first time?

— What if you talk to the pain like you speak to puppies in the park?

— What if you let the pain know that you are here, loving, caring
and kind?

— What if you consider your own life story when you feel a reason
to blame yourself for wrongdoings or mistakes?

— What if you honour your memories of what happened to you,
your fears and your helplessness as a child?

— What if you repair the damage, if you can, like you would repair
the bathroom door?

— What if you do what matters to you, without allowing judgement
to stop you in your tracks?

— What if you show yourself the compassion you show your four-
legged friend?

— What if you look at yourself every day, just like you looked
at your puppy the very first time you met?

— What if ...? You might discover that, like your puppy, you
are beautiful, lovable and good enough just as you are.

You are so beautiful!

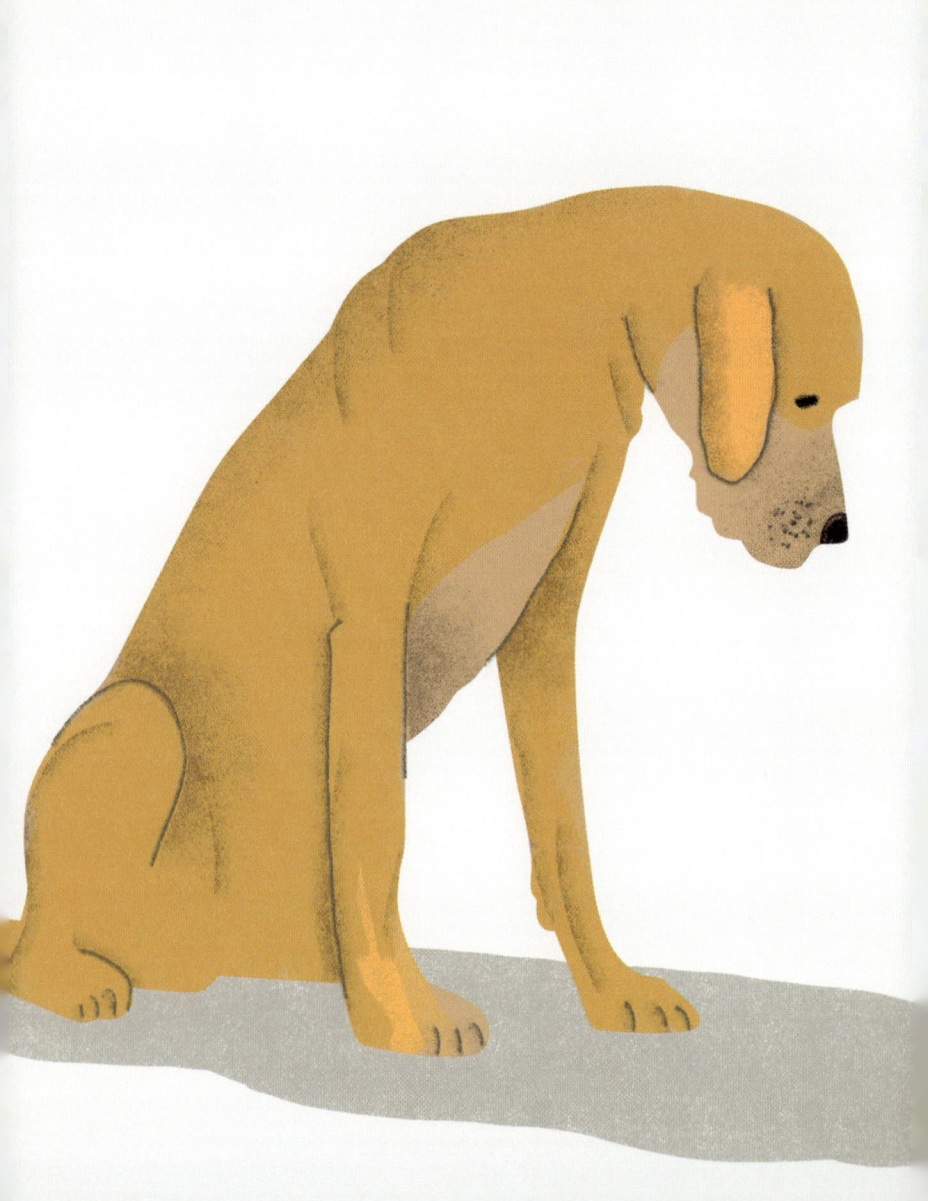

The truth and other stories

———————

A dog is a friend who listens with his heart
and replies with his tail and eyes.
That kind of communication is more powerful
than words. As long as you understand it.
Do you speak dog?

@cooper.thegs

Monty is a very special dog with very particular needs. She was left at a shelter and it was not easy to get her adopted. Being a mix of Great Dane and Dalmatian, she inherited the size of the first and the spots of the latter. A genetic predisposition also gave her, like many Dalmatians, deafness. She can never hear the postman coming or the food bowl being filled, and of course, she can't come when called. Shadows can scare her and fast movements are unsettling. And yet, she has found her forever home and could not be loved more. A special dog has found her very special someone. Or is it the other way around? Monty is a big dog, who fills a couch completely. She needs far more than half of a double bed where she snuggles under a doona, always ready for a pat and a cuddle.

If someone wrote a medical assessment of Monty, most of who she is would not be found there. The assessment would state the facts, including size, weight and her deafness and behavioural difficulties.

Imagine what this brief description would entail.

And now, based on what you read above, imagine with all your heart what the person sharing a bed with Monty sees when looking into her eyes. How do you think their heart jumped with joy when Monty learned to react to hand signals? Listing facts cannot describe the warmth in the owners' and Monty's hearts when both understand each other - without words!

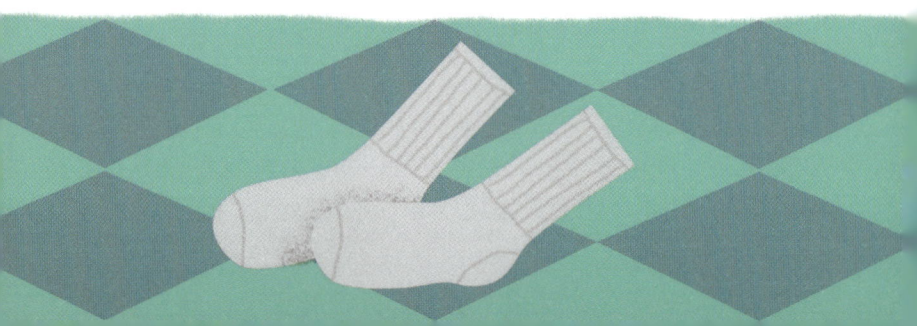

A story only listing facts will not touch you or make you laugh or cry, if you do not add your own experiences, memories, feelings, likes and dislikes to it. There are facts filed in your brain, but many more beliefs and opinions are stored and mixed in the same container. Your opinions, beliefs, memories and experiences all form a complex network and can have a huge influence on your decisions.

Does that sound complicated? If so, skip the theory and sit opposite your dog on the floor or on the couch. Look into her eyes and list some facts. Only facts; no feelings, emotions, memories or experiences you have created together. It's probably a short collection.

My list looks like this:

Dog, black, male, kelpie cross, four legs, one bent tail.

Does this say anything about who Amigo was for me? Or who I was for him? They are facts, but they do not contribute anything to sharing the special connection we had.

Now it is your turn again.

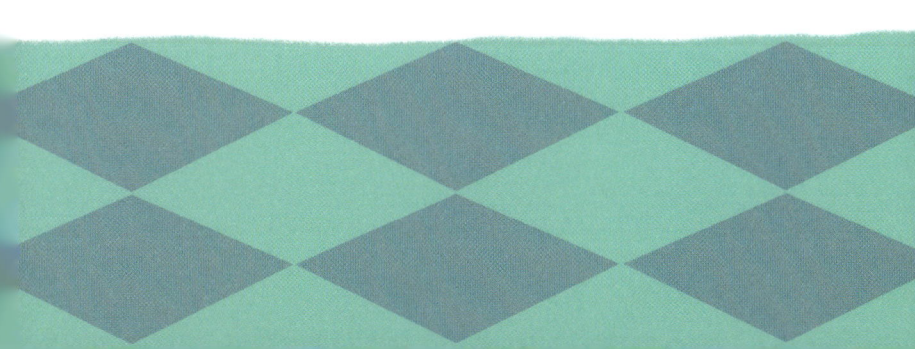

Look into your dog's eyes and let all words, thoughts and memories come that describe her in such a way that I could understand the special bond between you two, and how you not only see but feel her. The list would be endless, with each day adding more experiences and words to describe the bond.

No chapter would be long enough to cover all the little things I remember about Amigo. For one, there was the softer fur on his paw where he felt ticklish. Sometimes I couldn't resist tickling him there, and it made me smile watching the way he tried to stay close and move his paw away, a little annoyed but not enough to move. Some thoughts and memories are nice to have many times. It is helpful to more often recall those, relive them and go back to them again and again.

But not all memories or thoughts bring joy. Some are so painful that you would do anything to forget them. You might have tried, but I am sure you never fully succeeded. Trying to argue with yourself that staying with facts would keep the pain at bay hasn't worked either. Nor does blaming others.

In the boxed text, read about where it all started, and why we still try to think and work ourselves out of misery. If you decide that it is not the right time to read this, just move past it.

We formed a belief as a child that if we tried harder, if we could be better in anything or something specific, then we would be loved and cared for the way every child needs and deserves to be unconditionally loved every day. And sometimes being 'better', whatever that looked like in the eyes of others, brought us some relief and some momentary attention and praise. And so, we learned to work hard to change and to please others. We did not experience being good enough the way we were, so we don't dare to do what matters to us as adults, but instead are busy pleasing others. Social media, some friends, many books and blogs, leaders and gurus now continue trying to make us believe that we should change. They amplify the thought that it's the only way to receive love and acceptance.

Some of the suggestions you are bombarded with are not totally wrong, but they are not always helpful either. What is incorrect and totally unhelpful is feeding the false belief that if we 'better' ourselves, then we will be lovable and can love ourselves more. However, acceptance and love with conditions is never true love and never true acceptance. Unconditional love is what we all needed once, what your dog experiences every day and what you are worth too. Reach out to the child you were, with the same eyes and heart you use to see your dog, and let that child know that they were always absolutely fine just the way they were.

So, while some feelings, thoughts and beliefs make you happy and create a fuzzy warmth inside, others make you shiver, and fearful waves can touch the innermost part of you.

Have you noticed how quickly stories can take a turn, and how what started with a smile on your lips might have led to a clenched jaw and hunched shoulders. Maybe you have read the text in the box and memories came to the surface, and as much as you try, you cannot stop thoughts from appearing or emotions from being triggered.

You might judge me for leaving Amigo with the dog-sitter described in the previous chapter. You might remember a situation where you were scared for your baby. It is easy to feel overwhelmed, trapped or pulled in, and it is easy to start blaming yourself.

Your mind can do what the bird did to Amigo, which I described in the third chapter, when it landed on a wave and lured him into the ocean. I guess we can all relate to how this must have felt for this young, playful creature. All I could do was stand there and call him in vain.

Your thoughts can take you to a blissful heaven, but more often, they are like a rip controlling you. You are swept away from what you would like to feel and think, away from that peaceful place where you look into your pooch's eyes and soul and nothing else matters.

For some, rips might be difficult to imagine. However, most places on earth have, at least from time to time, torrential rivers carrying away whatever comes too close to the water.

Imagine your thoughts, beliefs, regrets and pain you carry as a torrential river. If you start thinking about something at 2 am, or when you are stressed, tired, angry or hungry, you are falling into the relentless current and getting carried away without a chance to step out or swim against the tide. Where are your rescuers, when the unforgiving rapid and relentless river of your own thoughts rip you off your safe ground?

A RESCUE PLAN: HOW TO FLOAT AND NOT DROWN

Remember Amigo and remember what all dogs do in tricky waters and breathe.

— Breathe out, breathe in and breathe slowly out again.
— Sit upright, with your feet on the ground.
— Get your most trusted companion on your side. It is never too early or too late to call her over.
— You are not alone; she is with you and you are with her.
— Put your hand on her side, feel her breathing and heartbeat.
— Notice your own breathing and heartbeat, or just continue to breathe slowly out and let the air flow back in.
— Focus on your arms and wiggle your fingers.
— Focus on your feet and notice where they are.

You will start to notice the ground under your feet again. Now you can continue in your mind, making the endless list of how beautiful your little puppy is and what she means to you. You have reached a safe sandbank. You have made it out of the river, however dangerous it once seemed to you.

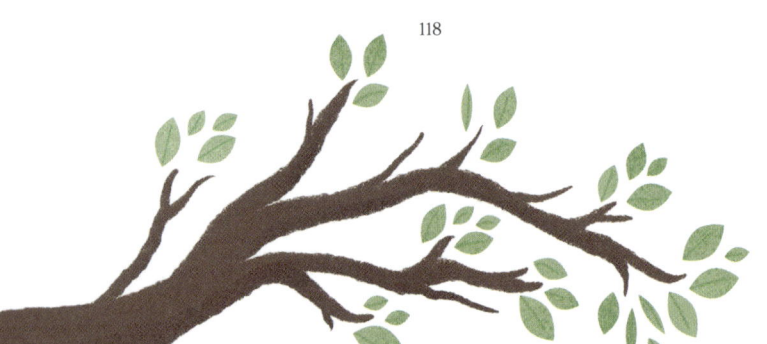

From the safety of the sandbank, you can look at this scary amount of muddy water full of painful thoughts. And from this perspective, you can start to let them pass down the river in front of you. You are not your thoughts. Thoughts are mental events, stories - facts or fiction - often painful emotions and traumatic memories. But all of this is not you. You are safe on the sandbank, with your trusted companion by your side. And from here you can see all that is bothering you floating down the river.

And it might happen that the sun comes out from behind a cloud, and there is a tiny sparkle on the river. Or you might feel a little nudge from a wet nose, letting you know that you stopped petting her and that she wants just a few more minutes of attention.

Take a thought for a walk

— What do you say to yourself while looking at your dog?
— How would you describe your dog to someone who doesn't know them?
— How many of these descriptors are facts? How many are beliefs, opinions or past experiences?
— Which of your thoughts would you label as helpful and which ones as unhelpful?
— Do you notice when you start holding on to unhelpful thoughts instead of letting them float down the river?

 Overcome your inner schweinehund

— Notice how thoughts, beliefs, memories and opinions make you feel. Pick one which is not too stressful and not too overwhelming.
— Notice what happens when you allow the thought – your own inner schweinehund – to drag you into a muddy, fast-flowing river.
— Notice how your inner schweinehund tries to pull and lure you in, and how it tries to splash you with mud and fill you with muddy thoughts until you might believe what they are telling you.
— Notice how you can choose to step back and how you can let the thoughts flow down the river.

You might even visualise the thoughts stuck on or in your inner schweinehund and floating down the brown current with it.

Keep in mind you are the one noticing and no thought can be bigger than you. You are the one standing and watching the muddy river of thoughts, and you are not the river. You are watching your inner schweinehund and its pull. You are not your inner schweinehund and you are not defined by it.

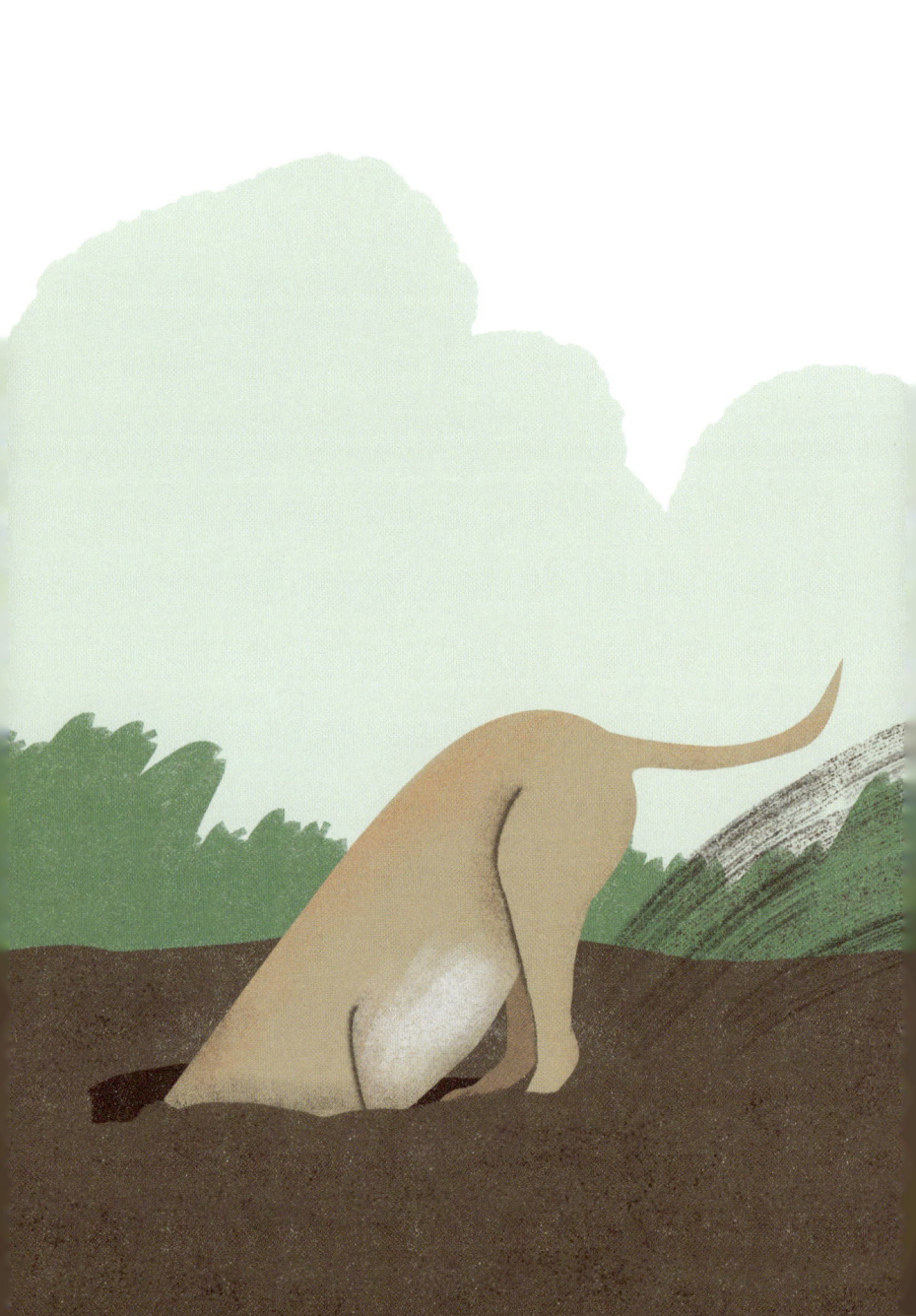

Just you and your fur baby

In the chaos of life, my dogs are my anchor, grounding me with their presence and unwavering love.

Alexandra Mahoney, Best Behaved Dog Training

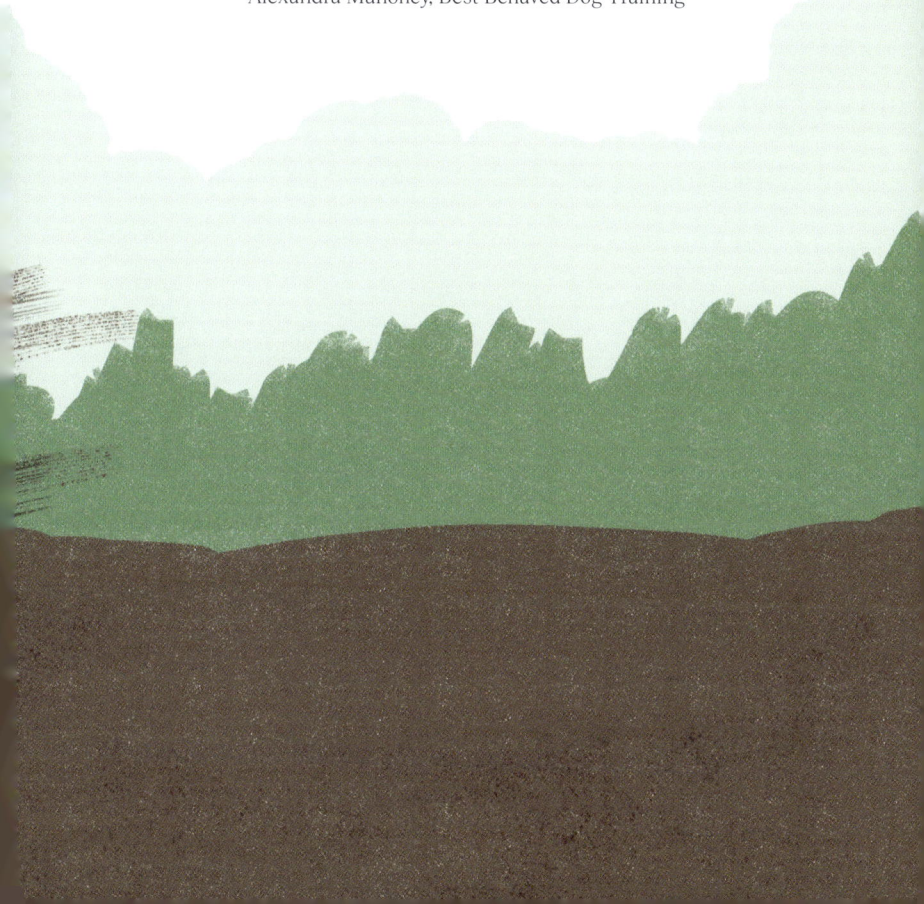

Dogs are the antidote to reality TV and social media. It is not surprising that the love of dogs and our relationship with them has changed. They have become important members of our households. In a time when we are flooded by people's ideas about how we should be and what is expected of us, they are a refuge of unconditional love and affection. Instagram and all social media are never telling the truth about how holidays really have been or how the night with amazing cocktails and photogenic food really felt.

Where is the respite? Some people have friends or family where they can just be, regardless of how much they weigh, if they have showered or are wearing appropriate clothes, but many people do not have these kinds of people in their adult lives. Maybe that would be okay if they had been unconditionally loved and accepted when they were little and started to make sense of the world, or if they experienced support when going through puberty, with all the trials and errors this time brings with it.

The judgment of those who should have loved us unconditionally is still felt, in the present moment or as a memory. And memories can feel like painful present moments too. All you have been through, and all you have missed out on when it truly mattered can get triggered in situations where you have to deal with other humans, the world or perfect portraits of people's lives on social media.

So you developed the hope that it would be different if you were different. You hoped that all would be better, if only you were better. Based on this hope and amplified by thousands of messages – many on social media – you told yourself that you could be happier, more loved and accept yourself if you ate less, exercised more, were prettier and had your dream job, or if you could be more motivated and find the miraculous power of confidence. However, regardless of the effort you put in, it still does not feel safe, because you can hear judgment, much of it in your self-talk. The world is still not safe and other humans can be wolves.

The only safe place for you now, without judgment, false pretence or disapproving looks, is with your dog. Maybe with the help of this book or a trustworthy human, you will discover that there is a safe place within yourself too.

In front of your dog, you can be the way you feel. You can cry or laugh; eat junk or salad; exercise or stay in bed. Regardless of whether or not you overcome your inner schweinehund, your dog loves you just the same, and with this unconditional love, your fur baby can motivate you to get out of bed and go for a walk.

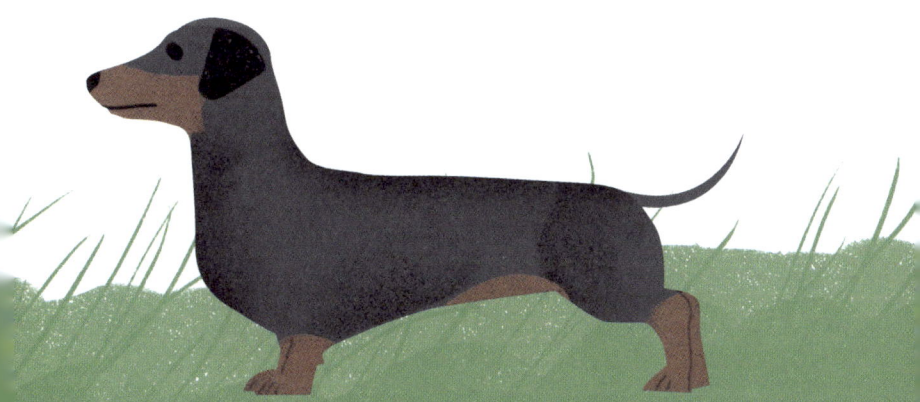

Your dog is the opposite of what you have endured from other humans. Comparison and judgment are not part of your puppy's make-up, and I think they are happier because of it.

When it feels difficult to escape depressive thoughts, something you can practice is imagining a small dog with curly fur snuggling close by your side, which might spark a glimmer of warmth and joy. A glimmer will not light your night or change your day or your life. Yet if you focus on a glimmer, you can get moments of warmth, which you can feel around your heart. Your breathing calms down and your thoughts slow down, too. A glimmer is not a magic wand, taking all pain away; it is a small warm light you can focus on while being in pain at the same time.

Just you and your fur baby, the title of this chapter, is an invitation to look at your dog, look into their eyes and feel the love they have for you, no matter what. Feel it in your body. Feel the love you have for them, no matter what. And if you can, open you heart and make room for this love to expand, making it possible to see and feel the first glimmer of how it would be if you loved yourself in the same way you love this four-legged miracle.

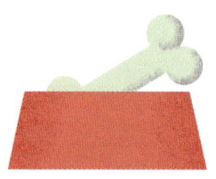

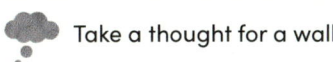 **Take a thought for a walk**

How does your fur baby spark a glimmer for you?

— Is it the ears, with the softest hair?
— The big brown eyes?
— The mouth, always looking like a little smile?
— The tilt of the head when you use some 'magic' words?

Choose one, focus on it and slowly breathe in and out.

Remember, this is an invitation and not a command. If it feels too challenging, just breathe out with a big sigh and put the book aside for another time.

If you do choose to focus on a glimmer, what do you notice?

Overcome your inner schweinehund

This is best practised at home, but definitely not when you are already overwhelmed and it all seems too hard.

If you feel well enough, dare to notice pain.

— Notice your pain, the one you hide from the world. Can you locate it in your body? If so, put your hand on that spot, wherever it is.
— Keep breathing. Focus on the out breath. And now, recall the glimmer you felt reading about the dog, snuggling with love and affection with their guardian.

Let your attention flow between the pain you feel where your hand rests and the glimmer and feeling of love – in the same way you would watch two dogs at the same time.

— What do you notice about the pain? Has it changed? Stayed the same? Has it softened?

The more glimmers you notice, the more you are on the road to creating a space where painful challenges in your life and the unconditional love you have for your dog – and maybe one day for yourself – can be there at the same time.

Self-judgments, the inner critical voice and disliking yourself profoundly are the biggest inner schweinehunds imaginable. But they can be overcome too.

Don't just blindly believe what I say, but don't blindly dismiss it either.

By daring to pay attention to your pain, you have already challenged and overcome a nasty, big and ugly-looking inner schweinehund. When you do so, it often changes its shape, its ugliness and its threatening demeanour. And by making room for a glimmer of beauty, warmth, hope and love, you have taken the first step to find all of what I invite you to experience inside yourself as well.

It is worth repeating: overcoming your inner schweinehund does not mean that you jump over this hostile-looking beast, afraid that it will turn around and bite you on the ankle. Overcoming your inner schweinehund leads to a different relationship with it. You stop fearing it, avoiding it and wasting time trying not to think about it. You acknowledge its presence and commit to overcome it. And so, it loses its power, changes its threatening demeanour and can become just a dog with a face like a pig.

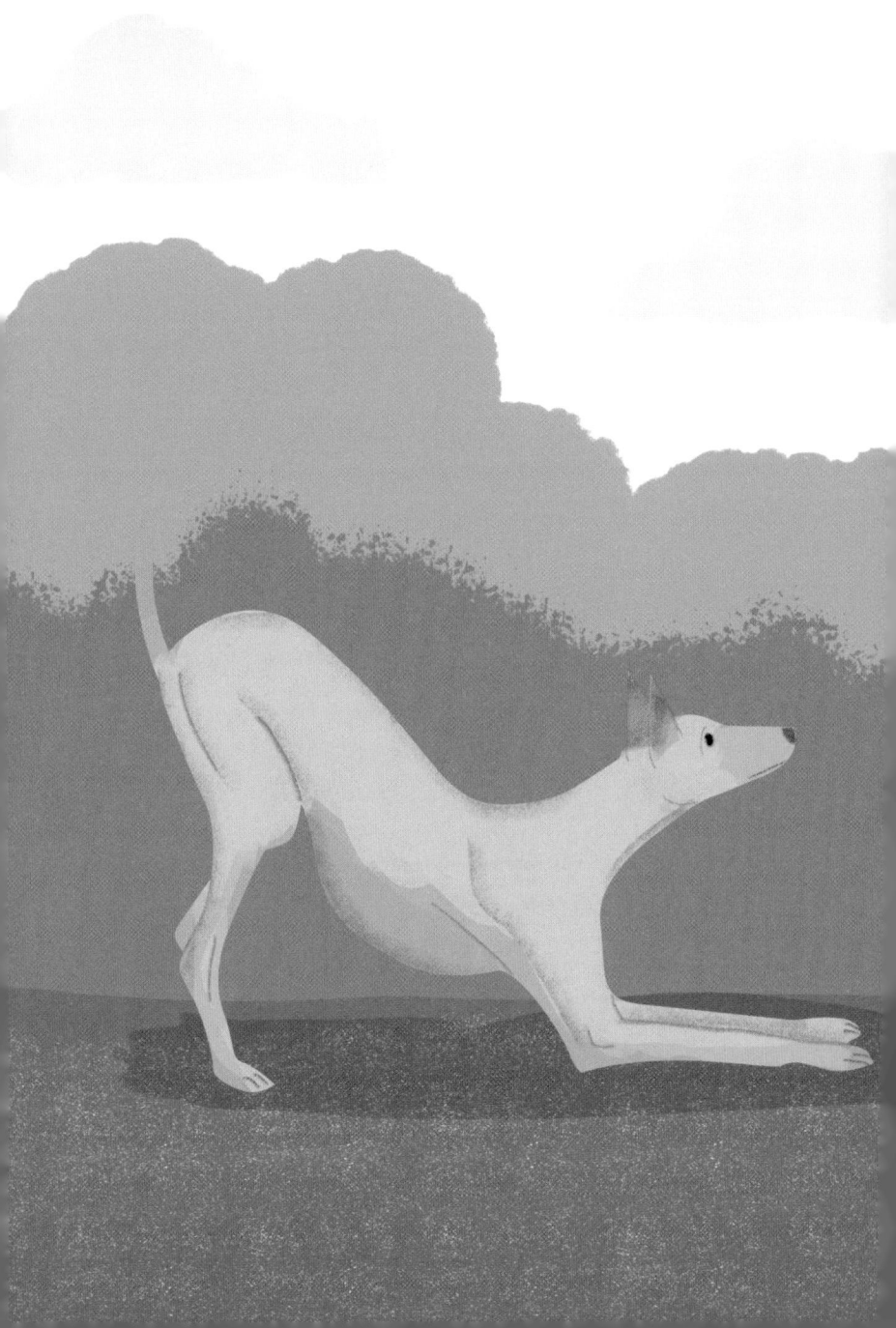

Through their eyes

Be the person your dog thinks you are.

C.J. Frick

The few steps taken barefoot on a carpet between the bed and the bathroom wakes Sugar up. Regardless of the time, she knows that the day has just started.

What is the first thing Sugar does? It is not switching off the alarm on a mobile phone and going straight to check social media and the news. She does not care what the weather is going to be or if the share prices in the US have risen or fallen overnight. What you can see, if you take a moment to notice, is Sugar getting up, stretching one leg after the other, rounding her spine and letting the tension go. Colloquially called a cat-cow pose in yoga (and *Chakravakasana* in proper yoga language). It improves posture and balance and also helps with back pain.

Amazing what Sugar knows and does, and equally amazing how often we know and choose not to do something that would make a difference.

Why? As mentioned previously, humans often do what gives them an instant sense of reward, the feeling of safety or the promise of less discomfort. So, checking the phone seems to give you more pleasure, or it seems to be more important than joining Sugar on the floor.

Sugar continues her morning routine with a bit more stretching and finishes it with a quick shake of her whole body, while she hears her human companion moan on the way to the bathroom and sees them pulling a face of disapproval when they catch sight of themselves in the mirror.

I am sure that Sugar has no idea what the disapproving look is about. From her perspective, the sun starts to rise with your appearance and she welcomes you with a wagging tail in the kitchen. It's a new day and a new start.

If the day begins with enough time for coffee or tea and a pat on her back, she settles next to the table for breakfast and enjoys the moment. If the alarm was set too late, no pants would fit and the phone is sending one 'ping' after the other, Sugar may get restless and stay close, hoping for attention. Or she may retreat to her mat, resigned to the fact that today is one of those days where she is not seen, heard or acknowledged.

If Sugar could speak, I assume she would ask, 'Why do you humans do to yourselves, what you would not do to your dog?' She would likely wonder why it is more important to check world news than to stretch your body. That your body, the home of health, physical and emotional wellbeing, gets less attention than a faraway row of numbers or a dinner someone else had last night would leave her puzzled. Maybe it is indefensible.

Going to her mat when things get hectic is Sugar's way of practising self-care. When Sugar was younger, she followed her human around the house, getting more restless and unsettled. When hectic takes over the morning and anxiety leads to frantic dashing from wardrobe to bathroom to bedroom to kitchen, when swearing, huffing, puffing and banging of doors is what Sugar witnesses, it can signal potential danger to her and can lead to 'co-escalation' (a mutual blow-up).

An out-of-control, anxious, stressed human can make their dog anxious and stressed as well. Sugar may give up hoping to be noticed and in her distress, settle on her mat. Similar to a child who isn't listened to and has to endure fighting parents.

So it makes sense to consider what your dog sees when looking at you. It can encourage you to make changes to calm your dog by calming yourself. Dogs learn from experiences even more so than adult humans do. Dogs learn from what they see and feel, exactly like you did when you were a young child. They, like young children, lack the ability to think through concepts presented with words. And while humans often define their superiority over animals with their ability to talk, anticipate the future and think through theoretical constructs, these abilities are actually their biggest source of pain and misery too.

In other words, instead of checking world news or social media first thing in the morning, you could join your dog in doing some stretches and some deep breathing before the day begins. Imagine the surprise on her face if you started the day relaxed.

Take a moment and notice how many of your fears and stresses are not happening right now, but are thoughts about the future or the past. Of course I do not know which of them are true, but what I do know is that the future is not happening right now.

Notice thoughts coming up and while you let them come, put a little sticker on them, labelling them in your mind as either 'helpful' or 'unhelpful' in this present moment. If you are unsure which label to use, take your dog's perspective and ask the question again, through his eyes. Ask him, 'What do you think is most important for me right now?' or 'What do you suggest would be the best thing to do in this moment?' Listen carefully to the answers.

It is not easy to look at thoughts. Some are created by memories and come with emotions. Often painful emotions. No memory is ever truly forgotten. Situations you survived before you could speak are stored in your body. Many humans I have spoken to find this a strange thought. They will tell me that they were far too young to remember, that the body is clearly not a brain and that their brain only came to life when they started to talk. Some hold the belief that what is really important is what happened or didn't happen to them later in life, so they focus on things going wrong around them or people being disappointing now. But when you ask yourself when you have felt like this before, you will remember. And most likely, this question will take you back many years from now.

Your dog will notice when you start making room for painful memories. She will feel the difference between you trying to distract yourself by cleaning, running around and checking your phone every minute, and seeing you take a heavy blanket and wrap it around you, stroking her calmly while being with her and all there is in that moment. 'It's not that easy!' I can hear you say. And I know it isn't. Sometimes attending to yourself, even just for a few minutes, can improve your whole day. Sometimes, you might not make this choice and a part of you sinks its teeth into a rope, where all your pain, shame and guilt are twisted into a thick piece of indestructible material. You are pulling like a Staffordshire bull terrier, a dog breed affectionately called staffy. Most staffies will not let go and can even be lifted off the ground, with their teeth tucked into a rope. If her owner takes a few steps back, the dog will follow. The tug of war will not stop. Both owner and dog are fully absorbed by the game.

The part of you that cannot let go ruminating and pulling is like a staffy with seemingly endless energy. However, you also have a part in you that is like the owner. They can pull the rope, engage in the game, step backwards, sidewards and even lift his dog. They can also decide to end the game by putting down the rope. And when they do, their muscly bundle of energy runs off and plays with other dogs.

While both were engaged in the game, nothing else mattered. While you have your teeth sunk into your worries, what ifs and your past wrongdoings and failures, nothing else gets attention.

While you cannot stop the thoughts from appearing, you can decide to stop pulling, just like you decide to end the game when it is time to go home.

Human minds are constantly busy and love to repeat what they have thought and done before. In this regard, I expect your mind to be like mine, coming up with doubts, scenarios and seemingly good arguments for staying engaged in the struggle. Many 'buts' and 'what ifs' are the result of a busy mind doing what minds do – throwing up ideas to protect your safety.

For some, the feelings are so deep and lead, again and again, to such a sense of unworthiness that they cannot notice any change when putting down the rope. I call this feeling shame, not to be confused with guilt. Shame is the result of what happened to you, the outcome of what you lived through when someone with more power than you made you feel unworthy.

If it is not too triggering, notice a thought or belief you cannot put down. Try to go back to where and how it was created. Listen to who created it first, and feel how you felt then.

Someone with more power did not keep you safe or an out of control situation threatened or destroyed your safety. The painful outcome is often not to feel worthy of anything good, or not to feel good enough regardless of what you might try.

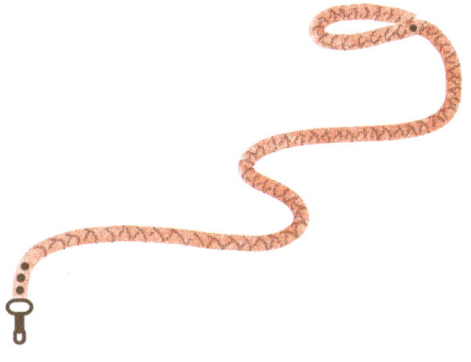

Through their eyes

Like some dogs who are unable to let go of the rope, you hold onto shame and feel it is your fault for not being able to 'move on'. Instead of blaming, yelling, pulling and arguing with the staffy, imagine staying calm and letting go of the rope, just like the owner did.

You can remind yourself that inside you is an undestroyable and strong self that has helped you to survive. This self can help you let go of the rope, step back and see the pull of shame for what it is – a reminder that something was done to you.

Shame needs to be held like you held your puppy for the very first time. Go back to that chapter on page 101, or just take a moment to hold yourself and your shame the way you held your puppy.

Guilt is different and a reminder of wrongdoing. There is not one living, thinking creature who hasn't done something they would not do differently given a second chance. There is no human who has not failed their own standards.

While shame sits deeper and affects the whole being, we will look at guilt in the next chapter. It can be painful too, and more pain is added if we refuse to forgive.

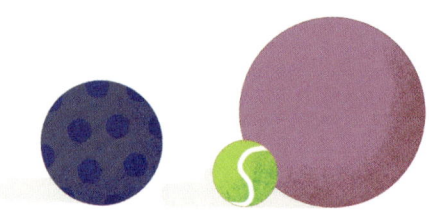

Take a thought for a walk

— What is the 'favourite' thought you get stuck into?
— Can you notice which thoughts are starting a struggle?
— What are you struggling with?
— For how long has this been going on?

 Overcome your inner schweinehund

Please be aware that some of the following points will talk about childhood, and it might remind you of your own.

— What happened when you stopped pulling the rope?
— How did your shoulders, arms and hands feel when you let go of the toy?
— Did you notice then that you could see other dogs playing and your dog playing with them? Maybe you were having a chat with another fur parent?
— Notice your thoughts telling you that it is your job to pull.
— Notice, as tricky as it is, what happens when you do not engage with your thoughts but do something else that makes your heart sing.

Decide on doing one thing that matters to you instead of thinking the same thoughts again. The thoughts might still be there, but you have decided not to engage shoulders, arms and head in pulling the rope but to relax and do something else instead.

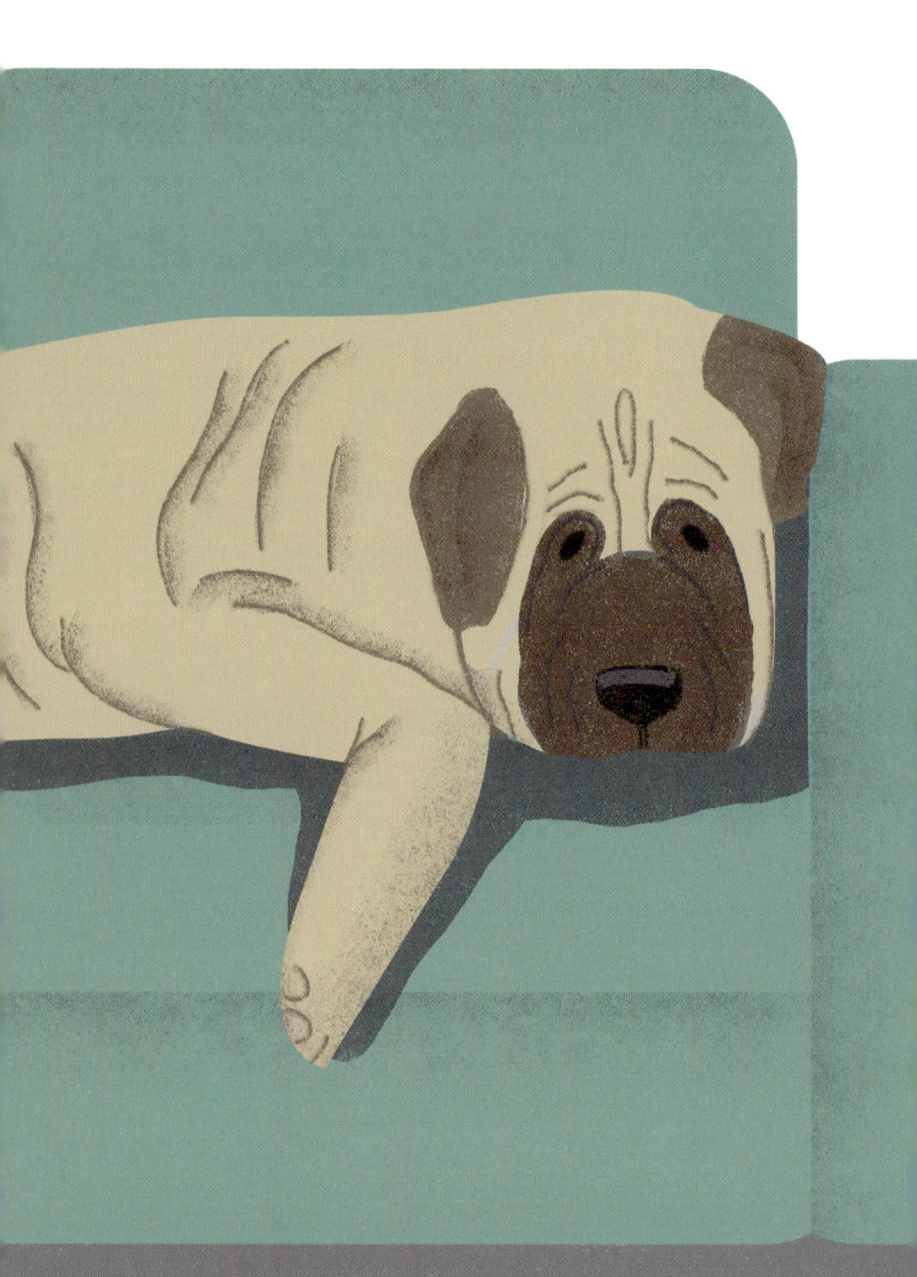

You are such a hobbledehoy!

The world would be a nicer place if everyone
had the ability to love as unconditionally as a dog.

M.K. Clinton

Living near a beach where dogs can run free, I have often seen the moment a little puppy is let off leash for the first time. Photos are taken and after a few steps away, the fluffy ball of joy is called back with the sweetest voice and welcomed with visible excitement – with cuddles and puppy treats.

While a puppy will occasionally run away, she will also learn that coming back to her two-legged friend is safe and a very happy moment for both. Dogs want to love and be loved, and so she will come more often and learn that obedience is a way of living in peace and safety.

Sometimes, something else is more important, and a dog, like any person, can get lost in the moment. Sniffing a tree or chasing someone else's ball takes the attention away from the recall. At home, and with less distraction from other dogs and less to sniff and get excited about, training leads to quick learning. Dogs are amazing at figuring out if it is okay to sleep on the bed or jump on the couch, or their mat. They can even read the room and adapt their behaviour, and clearly, they will remember different rules with different people.

Yet, there are still some rules that are more tempting to break than others.

Archie the labrador loves food. Of course he does. He also loves anything else that smells good – according to his taste – like socks. Archie taught his sock-wearing companion very quickly and successfully not to leave them lying around on the floor. After he found them in a laundry basket and was caught chewing one through

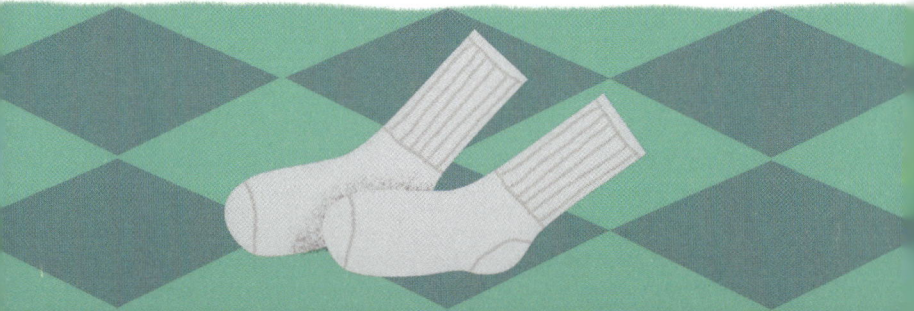

in a corner, socks were treated like muffins and the basket went up on a shelf. Archie is a clever dog, and he knew that he had plenty of toys for chewing and that there were other things better left alone. Following this rule seems to come easy after a few trials and errors.

One afternoon when his owner came back from work, Archie didn't run to the front door and wasn't seen wagging his tail and begging for food. He was in the kitchen. He walked slowly towards the door and had his tail between his legs. Of course, he couldn't respond with words to the question asking what he had done. When he made no eye contact, he was judged guilty and was let outside. Left out in the garden for a while, Archie was seen eating some grass and walking in a circle. That was very concerning and, minutes later, Archie was on his way to the vet.

The vet did some checks and suggested an ultrasound. When the vet asked, 'What have you done?', again the tail went between his legs and he avoided eye contact. By now, he looked really unwell. Based on past incidents, the vet suspected that he had eaten something he shouldn't have.

The ultrasound proved him right; there was something stuck in his stomach with a part trailed down the intestine, and the bowel was not able to pass whatever it was. This is called a linear foreign body and requires immediate surgery - costly and with some risks. Archie went through the procedure and a dishcloth was successfully removed. The bill was high. Archie had clearly done the wrong thing, knew better and should have made a different choice.

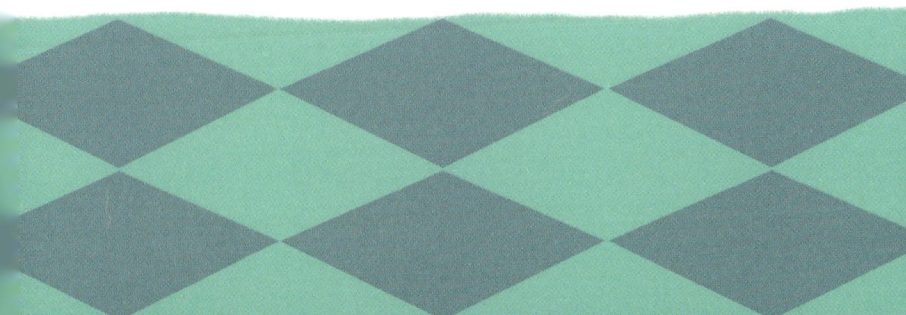

Without a huge mental struggle and without having to consider it for many weeks, months or years, Archie was forgiven for his failings even before he went through the vet's exit door. He got extra cuddles, love and care to heal and forget about the ordeal he had gone through.

Seeing the dog you love suffer will soften your heart and forgiveness comes easy. Do you agree? If so, how come you can be deaf to your own suffering and cold-hearted about the pain you feel after you have done something wrong?

I am talking about guilt. Guilt is defined as a feeling associated with doing something you know or should have known is wrong. So Archie is guilty, yet his suffering softened your heart.

Maybe he forgot that he is not allowed to jump on the kitchen bench and take something out of the sink. Perhaps you also forget the best course of action at times when you do the wrong thing to yourself or others. Is forgiveness connected to the amount of suffering for the culprit? In other words, do you forgive Archie because the pain he felt was his punishment?

Dansk is a Broholmer, also known as a mastiff. They are large dogs, bred for deer and wild boar hunting, and they also serve as guard dogs on estates and farms. The Danish Broholmer has a gentle nature and does not show aggression. Dansk follows his guarding duties and keeps his loved ones safe by placing himself between them and strangers, potential threats and unknown dogs. Dansk loves children and children love him. Due to his size and weight, he has had to learn to be careful and to stop when told to.

One day, when Dansk was already a mature dog, he trotted off exploring the park where he often went. He sniffed, walked and explored it with such enthusiasm; it was as if he had never been there. His human minder watched him and also saw a group of small children playing a bit further away. To make them feel safe, Dansk was called back, but instead of coming back, or at least slowing down, he went galloping towards the children. He ignored his name being called loudly, and when he reached them pushed a toddler, who got a fright and fell backwards. Shortly after, the leash was clicked to his collar and he was pulled away. A loud voice made it clear that he had failed in that moment and that he had clearly done the wrong thing. A few humans had an interaction with words, apologies were made, the toddler checked and an ice cream promised. There was anger, embarrassment and the afternoon in the park was suddenly ruined. Dansk was on his way home much sooner than planned.

Yes, there was anger and disappointment but also fear that this might happen again. Dansk went to his mat, and the human kept stewing and thinking about strategies to prevent a repetition.

Night was usually the time to enjoy some cuddles on the coach. Dansk walked slowly towards the place where he was used to spending the evening. And he could see, feel and smell a hand reaching out to him, patting him and letting him stretch out on two-thirds of the sofa as usual. Dansk was forgiven before the sun had sunk into the sea.

The next day was treated as a new beginning. It seems easy to forgive a dog, even if there are some scary moments, potential significant harm and an embarrassing situation in the park.

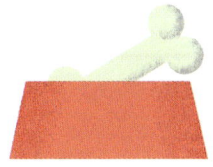

You are such a hobbledehoy!

There are many sayings about the importance of forgiving ourselves and to make room for the fact that we are not perfect. Some of these sayings suggest that all one has to do is to forgive in order to be free and move on. Often quotes advocate for forgiving others, which I believe is one of the hardest things to do and cannot be forced, suggested or pushed.

Self-forgiveness and self-compassion invite you to reach out with love, kindness and care towards yourself. Many find this a very new, strange and rather frightening concept, in the same way it might be new, strange and frightening for a dog who has spent months in a Lost Dog's Home to be led to a car. Nobody who cares would expect the dog to just jump in.

When I picked up Amigo from the Lost Dog's Home, we unlocked his kennel door, and I waited together with one of the carers at the door until he came towards us. We then spoke to him to start the journey of building trust. Trust doesn't just happen. Trust in yourself needs to be built, just like you built it with your dogs when they came into your life.

When we put Amigo on a leash, we did not expect him to immediately start walking beside us. When we want to teach a dog something new, we make sure to break it down into small steps and set the dog up for success. The steps must be small, yet still provide a little challenge.

We have memories on endless repeat stored in our brain. The internal monologue often starts with 'I should have', 'I could have' or 'If only I would have'. And at times, you remember situations where what you did was definitely not right. If Dansk had your kind of memory, he would have to acknowledge that what he did to the toddler was wrong.

We remember and know that we could have done better and that what we did might have hurt others. In hindsight, we see other options. We cannot go back and undo what we did, just like what was done to us cannot be undone.

Amigo had experienced the abuse, and he had to live with the fear of enclosed spaces, loud noises and a broken tail. Yet a happy life was possible, as he, like all dogs, lacked the ability to blame himself. While Dansk and Archie were both truly guilty, a new day was a new beginning for them.

Humans don't do 'new starts' that easily. You will blame yourself again and again, while at the same time not feeling one bit less guilty. You might punish yourself or have been punished by others for what you did, and yet the guilt does not shift. Feeling guilty after doing what you could to make repairs enhances the suffering. Blaming yourself endlessly does not make your life better or wipe out the feeling of guilt.

You can decide to start seeing yourself the way Archie and Dansk were seen by their human families. Yes, they had done the wrong thing. They had suffered or were corrected and helped to do better. And then they were forgiven. They had suffered enough and were worthy of a new start, love, care and connection.

Forgiveness is not an act that can be done and then ticked off the list of things to do. It is a way of being with yourself. It is a way of talking to yourself, noticing the tone and use of words and adjusting them. If you are unsure of what to say to yourself and how to approach yourself, just recall how you talk to your dog, and use similar words and a similar tone with yourself.

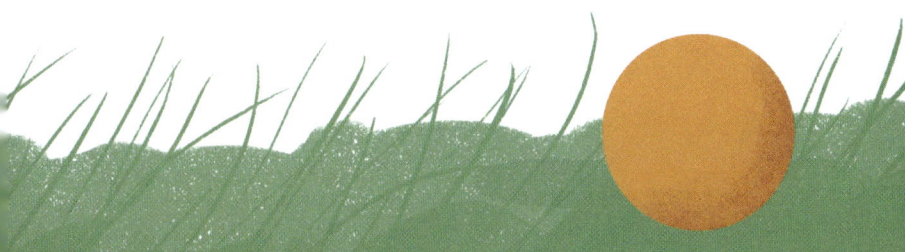

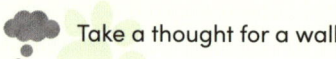

Take a thought for a walk

Notice how you talk to yourself and how you talk to your dog. If you talk more nicely to yourself than your dog, apologise to her and promise to do better.

If your dog hears the kindness and love you have inside yet you hear mainly the blame and self-judgment, then I invite you to change it and see what happens.

— How do you motivate yourself? How would you motivate a dog struggling with similar circumstances?
— What kind of words do you use when you describe your own mistakes? Is this helpful – or not?

Because you get so used to your self-talk, notice this on each walk for at least a week or two. If you hear internally a stern voice and see in your mind a task master with a raised hand, pointing finger, disapproving look and high demands, remember that it is you who can make room for other voices too. There are many voices inside you and you can choose which one to follow or not.

Even after one or two weeks of taking 'How do you talk to yourself?' for a walk, don't forget this question and continue to notice it as an ongoing practice.

Does your self-talk change between morning and night? Sometimes, getting tired or being hungry or upset leads to less self-care, despite you needing it much more than when you are happy and at peace with life.

Have patience. Continue with kind and loving self-talk, supporting yourself and what you are trying to achieve. While writing these sentences, it saddens me to know that we all beat ourselves up and expect to learn something new while tired, sad or stressed. At the same time, we agree that our four-legged companions deserve patience, support and lifelong encouragement, while we make sure that they are fed and patted before we start teaching them a new trick.

Change your self-talk again and again, so that if your dog could hear it, she would be convinced you are talking to her.

Notice the difference it makes in your life!

You are such a hobbledehoy!

🐻 Overcome your inner schweinehund

This inner schweinehund is another nasty one and tricky to overcome. It insists on guilt and likes the ongoing and endless pain and suffering. Forgiving yourself does not mean to just let go of the past – as if that could ever be possible. Forgiving yourself is rather living better with what you have done and showing compassion towards yourself.

While we do not dispute that Archie and Dansk did the wrong thing, compassion made a new start possible. You might argue that they are only dogs. True! And also true that you do not eat dish cloths or push little children. But it is also true that without forgiveness, a new start is impossible. And a new start makes it possible to attend to what truly matters to you.

Undeniably it is easier for dogs to make a new start. This cannot mean more and prolonged self-punishment towards yourself. This is a reason for more compassion for the amount of suffering you have inflicted upon yourself, sometimes for *many* years.

Imagine yourself in a court room. You have acknowledged your mistakes and gone through them all. When the prosecutor gets up, they will proclaim each one of them again, often with exaggerations. In your inner court room, the same script will be read over and over again.

Now imagine a defence attorney, calmly standing by your side. When they have the right to speak, they point out your age at the time, describe the circumstances you were in, explain your motivation for doing what you did and find words for the pain and suffering you had and still carry.

Listen to your defence attorney and what they have to say. It is only fair after the prosecutor got all your attention for so long. Be patient and let them finish. Notice how and if it is more difficult to listen to the defence than the prosecution.

Finally, it is time for an independent, wise, caring and fair judge to voice their verdict.

After all the suffering and no benefit of more suffering, the verdict can only be to learn from your mistakes and to be set free; to live the life you were always meant to live. Forgiveness gives you chances and choices you maybe did not think were possible anymore.

The pain of mistakes made will still be there. However, the pain of useless self-punishment can end. This will help you to do what matters and to live the life you want to live.

Just like Archie, Dansk, Amigo and all the other dogs with faults and failings, you can start afresh too. There is no dog or human who has never failed.

That you have done something wrong, and that you feel pain and suffering is what connects you with all humans. You are not alone, but connected to every human being on this planet. Each breath is a new beginning and a new chance to live life according to what truly matters to you. Often this means more moments of happiness, not stained by repetitive statements from your inner prosecutor. It allows you to be free and full of joy in the knowledge and felt experience that you are connected with all that lives under the sun.

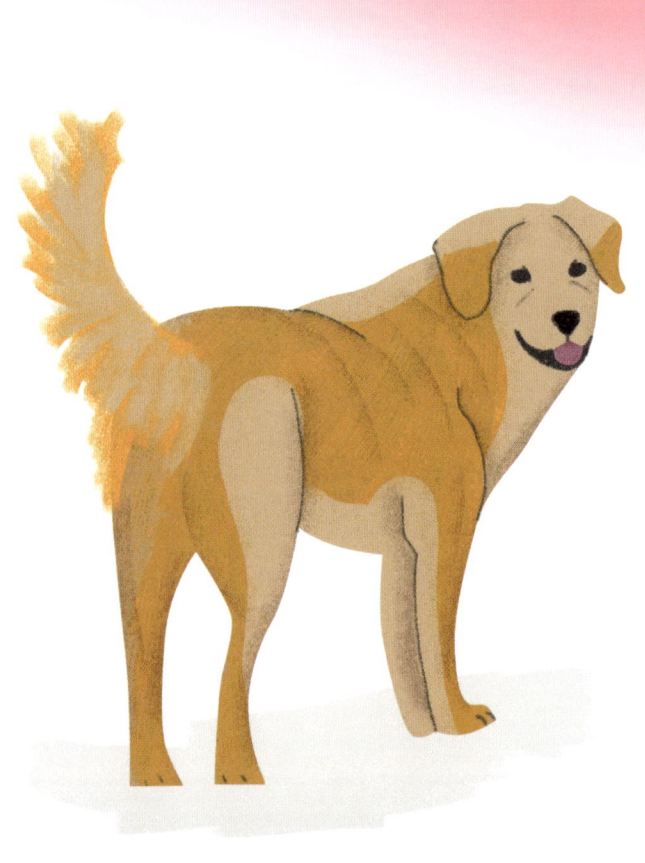

The hardest chapter

Like a bird singing in the rain, let grateful memories survive in time of sorrow.

Robert Louis Stevenson

A new beginning follows a loss. When your puppy was born, she lost the warmth and protection of her mother, and when she came to you, she left the closeness to her siblings behind and gained the excitement of exploring a new world. You might remember your puppy's restlessness during the first few nights, mourning the loss and adapting to the unknown. Your love and commitment to care for her was a new experience and needed her trust.

Losses and new beginnings are so closely connected that they can be imagined as two sides of the same hand. You hold what you love in your hand and at the same time you know that this hand will have to let go too. As nothing new can emerge without leaving the old behind, there is also no love without grief. If this is not the first dog in your life, you will remember how it felt when you had to say your final goodbye.

When you love, you risk being hurt when the love is lost. Some humans choose not to love again or not to trust, and this is an understandable attempt to avoid pain and grief. For you, with your four-legged friend next to you, this is not an option. Consciously or subconsciously, you chose to dare to love again, to give part of your heart to a creature whose only real fault is that they will most likely leave you before you leave them.

As much as you want to control all aspects of your life, you cannot control how long your trusted companion will be with you. You have heard of dogs with a very short life, and you have heard about the anguish when a puppy is farewelled before his life has truly started. You will have seen dogs trotting slowly behind their owners looking frail and old, but still showing up at the dog park day after day, for many more months than anyone thought possible.

Some dogs eventually go the way most of us wish to go one day – falling asleep peacefully and not waking up in the morning. For others, it is a painful struggle, and one day your trusted vet might ask you if you would like to consider ending the pain. There is no easy answer.

The magnitude of this decision is massive and not lightly handled. One part of you will scream to fight for one more month, week or day, while another part will feel the suffering and pain of a creature who once only knew excitement and could not wait to get out of the door and run freely.

How do you choose, when each choice creates or maintains suffering and pain? At times, your feelings are so torn and raw that you cannot trust them, as they flip from one side and one decision to the opposite, leaving you distressed and at a loss. However, inside we have a more stable tool to help us make a choice and to do what matters.

Your chosen values are a solid base, helping you to make the best possible decision. Your values are the same, regardless of whether or not you are feeling pain. Your values are the same if your puppy jumps with joy or your old companion has difficulty putting one leg in front of the other.

When you look at your dog and you know her well, you can see the world from her perspective and consider what is truly important to you at the same time.

As my dog Amigo got older, the champion in the dog park was beaten more frequently by others when chasing the ball. First my fast-legged kelpie cross was overtaken by border collies, then labradors. In the end, only dogs with no interest in balls were still behind him when he ran, then limped, in the rough direction of the ball. He still tried, and I felt that he had fun and didn't mind losing. It was always about the chase and never about the ball for him.

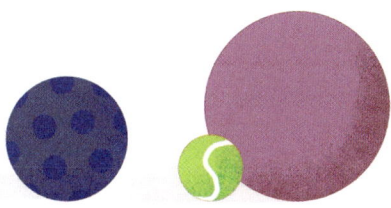

The hardest chapter

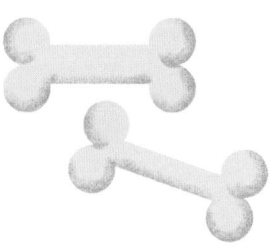

Then came the day when his back just failed him and he broke down, only to quickly get up and continue his walk. It happened more often, and the diagnosis was that this was a genetic disposition and that it would get worse. There were many days with slow walks and sunbathing in the backyard. Then there were more and more situations when his back legs failed him. Once, someone who witnessed it made a gasping sound, feeling the pain Amigo must have felt too. The once always bouncy and happy dog was finding it increasingly difficult to walk. He also developed more anxiety, got scared of himself in the mirror and started shaking when he heard noises he had not noticed before. Fun, adventure, freedom and being active - life qualities he enjoyed and pursued so much - were leaving his life, never to come back again.

These were his values, judged by what I witnessed over all the years he was with me. My own values towards him were stable and the same all his life - love, care and the commitment to do what was best for him.

The day came when relieving him of his pain and suffering was the best thing I could decide to do. It is never an easy decision, but looking back on it, I know why I made the right call and that it was based on what I thought best for him, and not just how I felt on a particular day.

And so he went peacefully, leaving me with the loss and inevitable grief. There is no magic way to deal with the pain of grief. There is no script and no right or wrong way. What can be helpful is to make space for it, and to allow yourself to go through all the feelings you have without censoring them.

Talk to people who understand, or talk to yourself in an understanding and caring way. Pat yourself, when you sit on the couch and miss the one who always enjoyed your touch. Sit there and tap your left shoulder with your right hand and your right shoulder with your left hand. Left, right, left, right, while you notice your breathing. Or just hug yourself and hold yourself tight.

Right after a loss, all your thoughts are dominated by it, and that is normal. You might try not to think about the loss, and that is normal too. Whatever you feel or think is welcome. It is best to make room for it, so that it can come and go without any pressure from you. If you close the door to the pain of grief, the pain will bang loudly and you will try tricks, remedies or distractions – ice-cream, lots of sleep or TV – attempting to drown the deafening noise. And even then, you will still hear the banging.

Remember that you were kind to your dog in pain, and you never told her how she should feel. If kindness was a value you chose to show your dog, it is also fair to embrace yourself with the same warmth you had for her.

Everything in my house, each walk and the park will remind me of the time Amigo was around. Giving his food, bowl and toys away was hard and made it so final. When your time to grieve comes, do it at your own pace. You might also like to keep some things, like a tag, a toy or, of course, all the photos on your phone. Whenever it feels right, create a place, maybe with your favourite photo of him and his collar or tag, and set some time aside during the day to mourn the loss and also remember the good times you had.

In a previous chapter on page 72, I invited you to create a peaceful place, a place where you can go to internally when things are tough. You can retreat to such a temporary resting place with the memory of your dog now at her final resting place. Make sure that you created one that truly fills your heart.

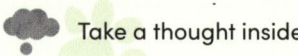 ## Take a thought inside

Instead of going for a walk with your four-legged companion, this time lie on your back or sit comfortably on your couch.

Remember a place you went with your dog, where everything was perfect. The weather was just the way you liked it. The temperature was not too cold and not too hot. The wind was not too strong, and the smell was your favourite smell in nature. It might have been the mossy smell in an old forest or the salty air at the beach. Recall what you saw and what you heard. It might have been birds or other people in the distance.

Remember what you did. Walking slowly, moving briskly or just lying on a blanket?

Visualise where your dog was and how she occupied herself. Sniffing around, walking by your side, snoozing peacefully ...

Give yourself time until you can recall the scene. When you can, start to relax your muscles on your forehead. Relax the muscles around your eyes and let go of your clenched jaw.

Let your breathing just come and go. Don't force it. If there are tears, don't hold them back. If there are no tears, don't wonder why and instead, focus on relaxing your shoulders. Pull them gently back to open your chest. Let the air flow in and out, while you continue to relax your stomach muscles. You might have to tense them, so you can feel the difference when you release them again.

Move further down and relax your hips and your back. A lot of tension is held in this area. Focus your attention on your hips, your back and all the muscles in the area and relax them.

Relax your thighs and your calf muscles. If you are lying down, let your feet flop sidewards. Relax your toes. Notice the steadiness of your breath.

Recall the peaceful place you started at and stay there for as long as you want.

If it is the right time, allow yourself to fall asleep. Otherwise, take a deep breath in and slowly exhale all the air from your lungs. Do this three times, before you gently get up and go on with your day.

 Grief is an inner schweinehund we cannot overcome, but only live with

Nothing will make the grief go away, but time might give you a different perspective. What the exercise above gives you is a strategy to live more calmly and wisely, and be more grounded.

And maybe one day you will dare to love again. In your heart is a place for many dogs. They do not compete for your love; the heart just grows bigger to make space for all of them.

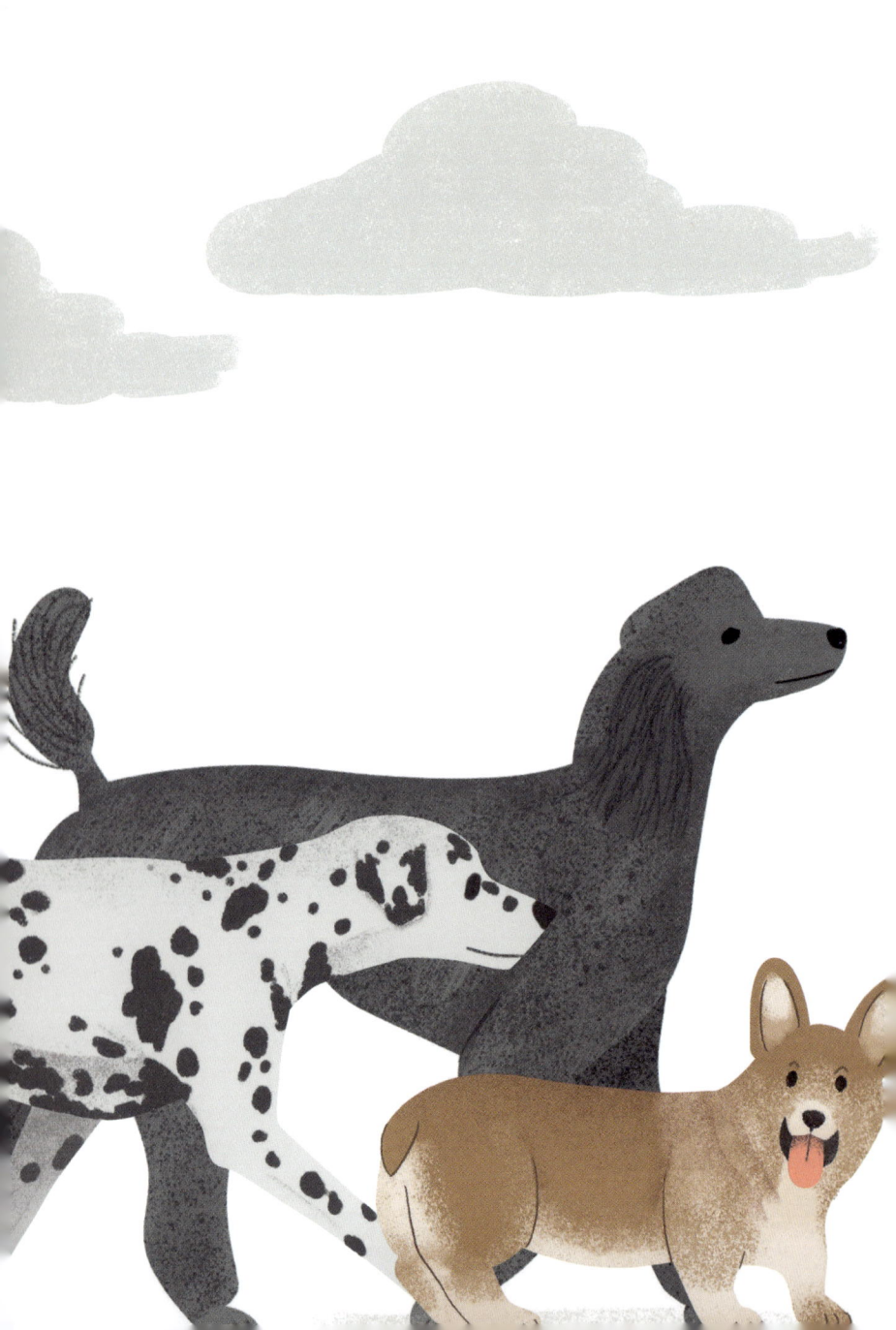

Make the coming week a special one

Changing your own perspectives, looking
at life through your dog's eyes and doing what
matters sounds simple. It is simple and not easy.

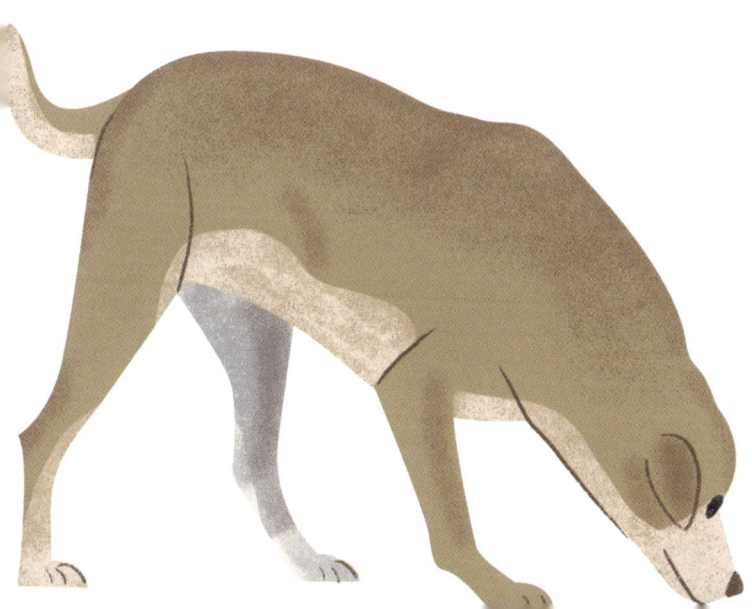

For your dog, every day is a Sunday. For her, the sun shines the moment she sees you, gets a pat, is fed or taken for a walk. For you, days can be without sunshine, and weeks can pass slowly or too fast. It all depends on your mood and the situations you face.

I hope this book has made you curious and ready to take on different perspectives and try new things, or it reminds you of helpful strategies forgotten far too easily. Maybe revisiting chapters in this book, or just committing to a week of the dog therapy outlined here, will help you to stay calm, curious and connected with yourself and the world around you.

SUNDAY

Be where you are. Right now, you can't be anywhere else.

Use the day to slow down, be in the moment, engage all the senses and just be. This last sentence is the exam hurdle of a master class in being. Most of us never pass!

As always, use puppy steps and celebrate an attempt as a success. Remember, you have some limitations compared to your dog when it comes to just being.

Try to notice whatever is around you and breathe for one minute in the morning. It can be listening to the birds and watching the curtain move, or observing the clouds in the sky and listening to your dog's snoring. Decide to do the same for two minutes in the afternoon. Set a timer or just observe two minutes pass on your watch. End the day with three minutes of noticing what is around you, gently pulling your wandering mind back to the present moment and breathing in and out. Take note of what you are noticing, and pay attention to the stories your mind is telling you in just the three minutes. Now imagine the number of stories you are exposed to in your mind every day. This is what makes creating a breathing and awareness space so important.

Your dog leads the way in 'being'. Try to follow for one, two and then three minutes each Sunday.

MONDAY

The playful child was told to stop and face the seriousness of life.
Now it is up to you to let them play again.

The serious part of the week might start for you on Mondays, when your alarm wakes you up – always too early. Or Mondays might be the same as any other day of the week.

Regardless, it is another day with another opportunity. You can use it to remember how you played as a child. What was your favourite toy? What did you enjoy doing? Observe how your fur baby plays now, carrying around a little soft toy and being delighted in the squeaky sound it makes.

What made your heart sing and be filled with joy? If you can, get a reminder of whatever it was, and place it in a spot where you can see and touch it. Maybe a children's book from the thrift shop? Or a little

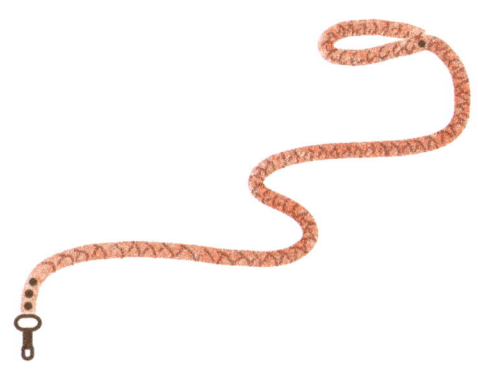

figurine reminding you of board games? Be creative and connect with the playful child full of ideas, dreams and potential that is still inside you, waiting to be allowed to live.

This token can remind you that joyful moments can be found and that playful moments without a measurable outcome can fill your heart with joy. As with all the other invitations, if you decline it, you will not find out if this can be true for you. And if it seems too difficult for you now, the invitation to try it will still be there next Monday.

TUESDAY

Embrace imperfections, like you embraced your perfectly imperfect puppy for the very first time. Hold yourself with the same kindness and compassion.

What starts with the best of intentions is often easily and quickly forgotten. It is not because you are superficial or bad; it is because just like your dog, you start to focus on the next challenge, on what is around you and what seemingly needs all your attention right now.

Like a puppy wanders off in the park and might lose direction, so does your mind. You might go back to putting yourself down, criticising yourself harshly or judging yourself and the world around you as never being good enough.

So, today's invitation is to notice if you have kept the promise you (hopefully) made, to talk to yourself the way you talk to your puppy when teaching her a new trick. You did not give up after the first attempt. You kept going. You showed persistence and perseverance, even if it took a while for her to get that weeing outside is highly appreciated, compared to a convenient wee on the carpet in front of the fireplace. All along your voice was firm but encouraging. Your words pointed out the desired behaviour, but were not used to put down or shame your dog and make her feel bad about her existence or for being a puppy.

Whatever new trick you would like to learn, whatever you might like to achieve – like walking more, watching less TV, contacting someone or learning to swim – the best way to get there is the same way you taught your puppy not to wee on the floor.

WEDNESDAY

One step forward is better than a thousand thoughts about moving. Happiness is not the reward for doing what matters. It is rewarding to do what matters.

This day can be a challenge – like any other day – but Wednesdays are right in the middle of the week, between the weekend too long gone and the faraway weekend to come.

Some people feel flat or flatter than usual on this day. However, this day is giving you another chance to choose. You now know some strategies that could make a difference for the better. But before jumping into any activity, or beating yourself up for not doing anything, start again by considering who or what is truly important to you.

You might feel the wet nose pushing against your knee, inviting you to pat or scratch her behind the ears. So, she is truly important to you, as Amigo was to me. The next step is to think about one thing you could do to show your best friend that she matters to you. Maybe it is time to bath her and watch the happy dance she does when shaking off the last drops from her fur. Maybe it is getting up and walking to the park, where she can run wild or watch other dogs from the sideline.

This is not a recipe to feel better or to make you happy. It is an invitation to do what matters and then to notice how you feel. Even if nothing or very little has changed for you, you can go to bed knowing that you made a difference in your dog's life, by giving her the extra attention and a cuddle and letting her run off some steam, before settling on the couch together.

What is one thing you could do for yourself, not based on what you should do, but emerging from what is truly important to you? Remember one small step forward is more helpful than one thousand thoughts about what makes it difficult and what might hold you back.

THURSDAY

A smile is a powerful way to improve your day and connect with others.

The main difference between humans and dogs is that they do not use words to communicate, yet we know how they feel, because of the many other ways they can express themselves. Their body and mind work closely together, and when they are happy, they wag their tail. Seeing playful dogs having fun can lift our mood as well.

Sometimes all you need to do is to go to a dog park and watch these creatures, tall and small, sniffing, running, chasing a ball or just lazily enjoying the sun or rolling in the mud. What your eyes see, your brain absorbs, and this can warm your heart and make you smile. It is another human superpower dogs do not have; you can make a deliberate choice to smile.

This Thursday, you can choose to smile with your lips and your eyes, while relaxing your jaw, each time you see your dog wagging her tail or trustfully looking at you.

Your deliberately smiling face can warm your heart and make a difference to your day. Don't trust my words. Try it out! Do not force yourself and, as always, use puppy steps. If a full-face smile is a step too big, start by relaxing your jaw and letting your tongue freely wander around in your mouth. It might sound weird, but invite yourself to experience how it feels with an open heart to either take a puppy step or do a big wide smile.

FRIDAY

In the dog park of your thoughts, let them chase each other, roll in mud and jump to conclusions, while you stand back and watch. Not one of them has the power or the control to tell you what to do.

Another difference between dogs and humans is that humans can have lots of thoughts at the same time. We are able to multitask, to a degree, and to multi-think, often to a degree that leads to exhaustion. Thoughts are racing each other and reappearing at a frequency and speed no film director could portray adequately in a movie. Any attempt would make your head spin and you would feel dizzy.

You will often feel like you have no control, rather like an object pulled, in first one and then another direction, thrown around and stretched until breaking point. Remember the first time you went with your little puppy to a dog park? Amigo was so excited to meet and greet all his new friends, and they were equally excited to sniff him. But there were so many legs and snouts and faces that he started to feel overwhelmed and signalled his submission by rolling on his back, the licking, nibbling and sniffing continued.

It didn't look like fun anymore, and I stepped in and picked him up. From the safe place of my arms, he could now watch the others run around and do what dogs do. Let's imagine that all these dogs are thoughts running around in your mind. You can try to control them, sort them, lock them up or try to ignore them. It will turn out to be an impossible task. There are still one or two not listening to your calls – a border collie jumping the fence and two pugs rolling in the mud. Just like your thoughts. However hard you try, they are not manageable in the long run. You can try to ignore them, put on dark glasses, turn around, get upset. The dogs, like your thoughts, are still running wild. The moment you wake up, switch off the TV, unpack your latest purchase or finish your yoga class, thoughts you tried to negate are back. They chase you like a beagle chases food, and no takeaway food delivery calms them down for long.

I invite you to take yourself in your arms, like I took Amigo, and observe your thoughts the way we observed the dogs in the park. We let them all be. We do not judge them, or try to control, manipulate or lock them away. By doing the same to your thoughts, you will discover that not one of them can hurt you, tell you what to do or ruin your day. You can watch them, observe which ones appear most often, notice what they are saying and, at the same time, keep a safe distance. With this new perspective, thoughts are just like dogs running wild. They do not have to make you wild as well. You are not them; otherwise, how could you watch them? You are as safe as Amigo in my arms, and from this place you can decide calmly what to do next.

SATURDAY

Your world will change if you forgive yourself the way you wholeheartedly forgive your dog, so many times throughout their life.

There is no week in our adult life when we have not made a mistake and become aware that we should have or could have done something better than the way we did it. Some of your mistakes might seem small to others, but you find them difficult to forgive. You might ruminate and go over the situation again and again, as if thinking about it could create a different outcome. You are not crazy for trying to figure out what went wrong and why. Your brain tries to help you, so you do not make the same mistake again. What your brain ignores at 2 am is that this exact situation cannot come back, and so you will not have the chance to undo what you did.

Your brain is not always helpful by insisting that you can learn to do better by endlessly repeating what you did wrong. You need to get out of this loop. The first step is to thank your brain for what it is trying to teach you, but it is also important to let your brain know that the

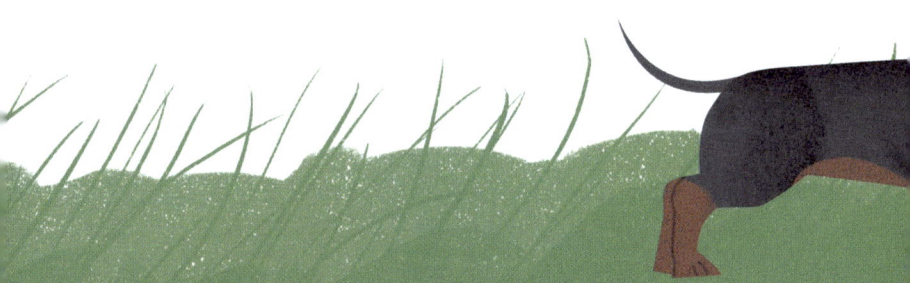

past will not repeat itself, and that as long as you breathe, you have a chance to learn from mistakes. Making the commitment to do better is totally different from trying to undo a past mistake by constantly thinking about it.

Remember the look on your dog's face after they destroyed something or were caught in the act? There is a willingness to do better and a sense that he has stuffed up. And this is where I invite you to treat yourself as you treat your four-legged best friend. Instead of endlessly repeating what you should have done or could have done, go to a mirror and look at yourself, as caringly and lovingly as you look into your dog's eyes in the morning. You might notice that this can take a while and might feel silly at first. Your mind comes up with excuses and laughs at this suggestion. Remember that your brain tries to protect you, and there might be the thought that what you see will not delight you.

Thank your mind for all its concern and walk towards the mirror.

Look into the face of this human who tries so hard - often harder than any dog - yet she treats herself with contempt and a harshness she would not accept in anyone, towards any animal. So many women, especially, are suffering trying to reach unachievable perfection.

Look into the eyes of this person who has grown up being told to be tough and not to show emotions. What would happen if he treated himself the way he treats his dog? So many men, especially, are lonely, because they are too afraid to share how they really feel.

What would happen if you could forgive your own mistakes, as you forgive your dog's, repair the damage and pay the bill? I believe your world would change, as your dog's world changed when your unconditional love, your care, your patience and your willingness to never give up entered their life.

Consider your week to be a mini version of your life. Maybe your days are a mini version of your weeks. The purpose of this book is to make you aware that changes are possible, and that you have choices as long as you live. Your four-legged best friend can remind you of choices that matter and can help you live a meaningful life. It does not mean that your life will always be full of joy and happiness, but it does mean that you can make deliberate choices to do what matters, not only for your fur baby but for yourself as well.

Has this book changed something in your life? Strictly speaking, the answer will be no. This book cannot change anything in your life, but doing what is suggested here can. So, if nothing has changed since you started reading this book, my suggestion is that you go back to the beginning and commit to actually doing the exercises, and not just quickly scanning through them.

Remember that the past is gone and will not come back. You might at times mourn it, at other times be glad about it. In both cases you can only access the memories. What the future holds is unknown, regardless of how much you plan, anticipate or think about it. The only moment you have is right now, so use this moment to enjoy what you can enjoy, and to appreciate the love and the trust your dog gives you without fail on any given day. Do the same for yourself.

Take a thought for a walk

Read the short phrase of the weekday and take it for a walk, with or without your four-legged companion. Let each of these quotes be your guiding thought for each day of the week.

 Overcome your inner schweinehund

After choosing to overcome your inner schweinehund many times, to embrace the discomfort of taking a risk, to look fear in the eye and to do what truly matters, you will find out that the schweinehund changes.

The massive, ugly, scary pig-faced dog that frightened you morphs into a fearful little roly-poly dog with a piglet's face. Not the puppy of your dreams, but a creature you can be with.

New schweinehunds will emerge and challenge you, but knowing what you know now and by doing what I invite you to do, they will go through a shrinking process, becoming a miniature that is unable to stand between you and a richer and more meaningful life.

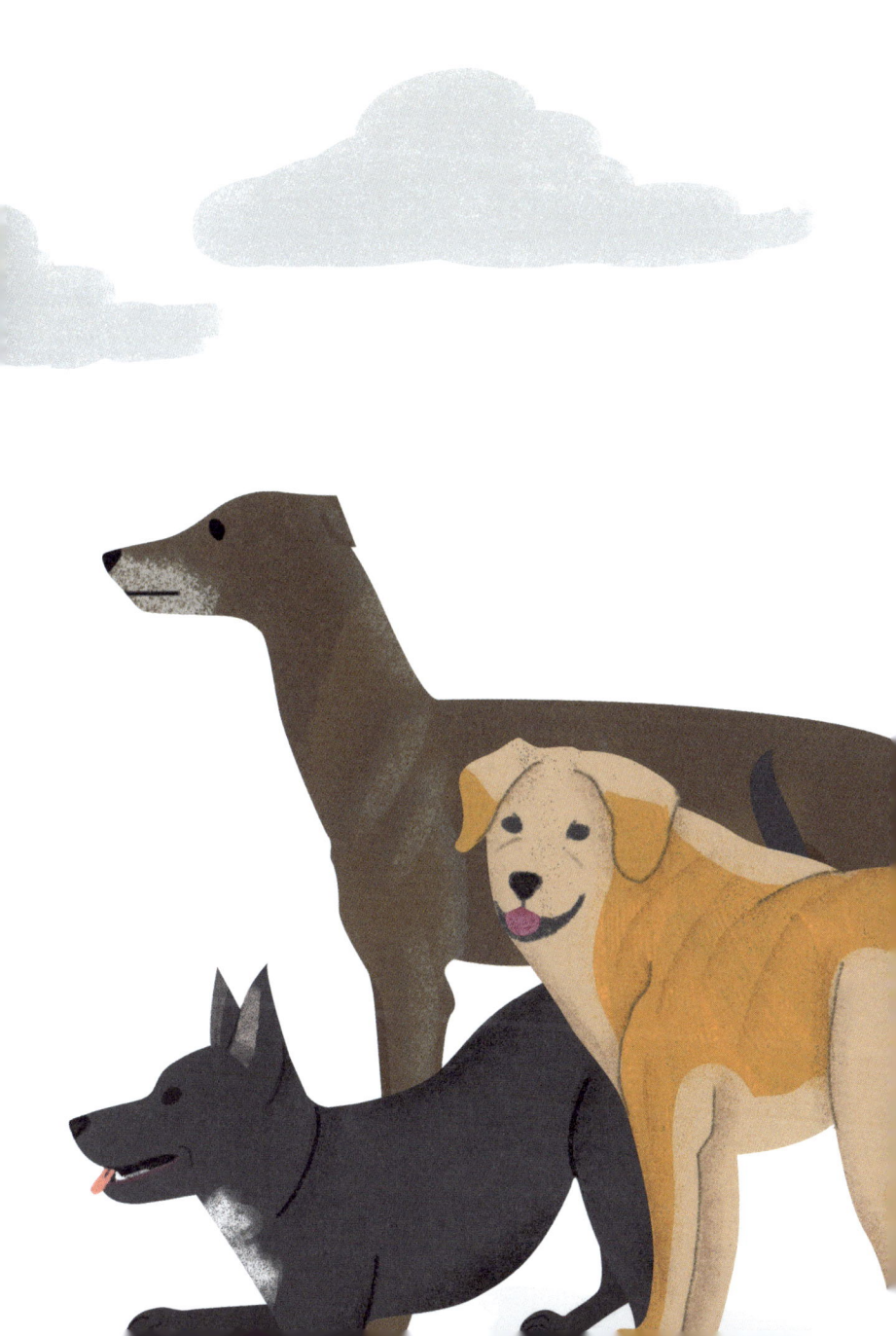

RESOURCES

It might be triggering to read through this list of resources. You might
have tried one of the suggestions and it has not worked for you.
That is hard, disappointing and painful. However, it does not mean that
nothing will ever help you. Rather, it means that you have not found
the right support yet. Even if you have given up hope, I hold the hope
for you and know that things can change.

The best resources are inside every one of us. They are always
accessible and free. To help you find them when you cannot access
them, contact:

Australia
Lifeline 13 11 14 www.lifeline.org.au
Beyond Blue 1300 224 636 www.beyondblue.org.au

United Kingdom
NHS 111 www.nhs.uk
Samaritans 116 123 www.samaritans.org

United States
988 Suicide and Crisis Lifeline 988 www.988lifeline.org

Or call any other helpline you have found useful before.

To build more resources, read about other people's experiences and
find useful metaphors (without dogs) read: *The Happiness Trap* by
Russ Harris. Check out chapter 25 for information on the difference
between values and goals.

On the following website under 'Free Stuff', the author shares with
unfailing generosity a variety of helpful resources, including videos
and audio recordings: www.actmindfully.com.au

For those fur parents who are also super-feelers, and are sometimes in pain because of being disappointed in relationships with other humans read: *Escaping the Emotional Rollercoaster* by Dr Patricia Zurita Ona.

If it made sense to you that you are worth the same love and care your dog is, but you struggle how to find a way to do that for yourself read: *The Mindful Path to Self-Compassion* by Christopher K. Germer PhD.

Of course, there are also a lot of different apps and audio books, if reading is not really your 'thing'. There are ACT-guided meditations to be found on the app *Insight Timer*. Search for Lou Lasprugato and choose one of the resources he donated to the app. For example:
'Treating Emotions as Guests'
'Responding Compassionately to Suffering'
'Being Here Now'
'Grounding and Centering' ... and many more.

Maybe you have tried therapy, or you are in therapy while reading this book. You might have been told, or knew all along, that part of your struggle is not because of what you did or did not do, but because of what was done to you. The feeling of being overwhelmed now was created when you were overwhelmed then and there.

This practical workbook is written by someone who has a lot of experience with and compassion for those in pain: *Transforming the Living Legacy of Trauma: A Workbook for Survivors and Therapists* by Janina Fisher, PhD.

Remember, whatever you feel, regardless of how big the pain is, you are not alone. Many people in a similar or the same situation will feel like you. You feel that way because you are human.

Pain and suffering is what all humans have in common, so when you take your dog for a walk and you see other humans, remind yourself that they know pain and suffering too. And maybe one day you can dare to trust one of them again, like you dare to love your puppy.

ABOUT THE AUTHOR

Angelika von Sanden is a Melbourne-based trauma counsellor, working mainly as a clinical supervisor. Her personal and practice's foundation is care, honesty and respect, using Acceptance and Commitment Therapy (ACT) and other approaches. She has a background in social work and a Master of Counselling. Fluent in German and English, she loves dogs, metaphors and a language free of professional jargon.

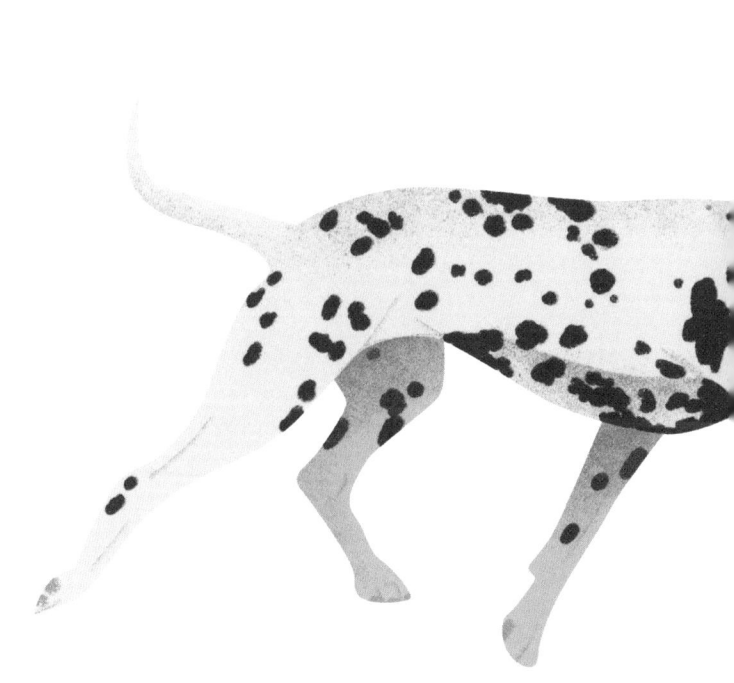

Published in 2025 by Hardie Grant Books,
an imprint of Hardie Grant Publishing

Hardie Grant Books (Melbourne)
Wurundjeri Country
Building 1, 658 Church Street
Richmond, Victoria 3121

Hardie Grant Books (North America)
2912 Telegraph Ave
Berkeley, California 94705

hardiegrant.com/books

Hardie Grant acknowledges the Traditional
Owners of the Country on which we work,
the Wurundjeri People of the Kulin Nation
and the Gadigal People of the Eora Nation,
and recognises their continuing connection
to the land, waters and culture. We pay our
respects to their Elders past and present.

Excerpt on page 15 from *A Lamp in the
Darkness* © 2011 Jack Kornfield used with
permission from the publisher, Sounds
True Inc.
Excerpt on page 65 from *Unbinding the
Heart* © 2012 Agapi Stassinopoulos used
with permission from the publisher,
Hay House LLC, Carlsbad, CA
Excerpt on page 89 used with permission
of Russ Harris, from *Act with Love* © 2009;
permission conveyed through Copyright
Clearance Center, Inc.

Every effort has been made to trace
copyright holders and obtain their
permission for the use of copyright
material in this book. Please contact
the publisher with any information on
errors or omissions.

 A catalogue record for this
book is available from the
National Library of Australia

Sit, Stay, Grow
ISBN 978 1 76145 110 2
ISBN 978 1 76144 320 6 (ebook)

10 9 8 7 6 5 4 3 2 1

Publisher: Tahlia Anderson
Head of Editorial: Jasmin Chua
Project Editor: Ana Jacobsen
Editor: Brigid James
Design Manager: Kristin Thomas
Designer: Claire Orrell
Head of Production: Todd Rechner
Production Controller: Jessica Harvie

Colour reproduction by Splitting Image
Colour Studio
Printed in China by Leo Paper Products LTD.

MIX
Paper | Supporting
responsible forestry
FSC® C020056

The paper this book is printed on is
from FSC®-certified forests and other
sources. FSC® promotes environmentally
responsible, socially beneficial and
economically viable management of the
world's forests.